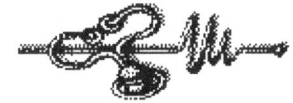 

A Glossary of Medical Terms

A B C D E F G H I J K L M N O P R S T U V W X Y ?

ACTH (Adrenocorticotropic hormone) -- Hormone produced by the pituitary gland. It stimulates adrenal glands to secrete the hormones they produce, including cortisone and cortisol.

ACTH (Adrenocorticotropic hormone) deficiency -- Too little ACTH produced by the pituitary gland; often the result of a pituitary tumor. Symptoms include weakness, fatigue and gastrointestinal disturbances.

AIDS (Acquired Immune Deficiency Syndrome) -- Major failure of body's immune system (immunodeficiency disease). It decreases body's ability to fight infection and suppress multiplication of abnormal cells, such as cancer cells. See Immunodeficiency disease. Caused by a sexually transmitted virus, contaminated blood or via the placenta to a fetus of an infected mother.

Abell-Kendall modification -- Modification of a lab test developed by Drs. Abell and Kendall.

Abruptio placenta -- Separation of the placenta from the uterus during the last trimester of pregnancy. **Abscess** -- Swollen, inflamed, tender area of infection filled with pus.

Achalasia -- Condition of the esophagus that disrupts normal swallowing.

Acid-base imbalance -- Imbalance that occurs when body retains too much acid or too much base. **Acidosis** -- Pathologic condition resulting from accumulation of too much acid in the body. **Acidosis, metabolic** -- Too much acid in the body due to loss of base.

Acidosis, respiratory -- Too much acid in the body due to accumulation of excess carbon dioxide. **Acromegaly** -- Condition that afflicts middle-aged people. Characterized by a gradual, marked enlargement of the bones of the face, jaw and extremities. Caused by overproduction of growth hormone by pituitary gland.

Acute -- Beginning suddenly. Severe but of short duration.

Acute intermittent porphyria (AIP) -- Disease of porphyrin metabolism. Symptoms include recurrent attacks of abdominal pain, gastrointestinal symptoms, neurological disturbances and an excess of porphobilinogen in the urine.

Acute pulmonary edema -- Set of dramatic, life-threatening symptoms, including extreme shortness of breath, rapid breathing, anxiety, cough, bluish lips and nails, and sweating. Usually caused by congestive heart failure. See Congestive heart failure.

Addison's disease (Adrenal insufficiency) -- Condition caused by inactive or underactive adrenal glands. Symptoms include weakness, low blood pressure, behavior changes, abdominal pain, diarrhea, appetite loss and brown skin.

Adenocarcinoma -- Any of a large group of cancerous tumors of a gland or gland tissue.

Adenoma -- Benign tumor of glandular cells. May cause excess hormone secretion by the affected gland.

Adhesions -- Small strands of fibrous tissue that cause organs in the abdomen and pelvis to cling together abnormally, creating a risk of intestinal obstruction.

Adrenal -- Pertaining to one or both glands located adjacent to the kidneys. These glands secrete many hormones, including adrenalin, and play an important part in the body's endocrine system.

Adrenal cortex -- Outer layer of the adrenal gland. Secretes various hormones including cortisone, estrogen, testosterone, cortisol, androgen, aldosterone and progesterone.

Adrenal hyperplasia -- Abnormal increase in the number of normal cells in the adrenal gland(s). **Adrenal insufficiency** -- See Addison's disease.

Adrenal medulla -- Middle part of the adrenal gland. Secretes epinephrine (adrenalin) and norepinephrine.

Adrenal medulla tumors (Pheochromocytoma) -- Tumors of the medulla, an inner layer of the adrenal gland, called pheochromocytomas. Tumors are rare and secrete norepinephrine and epinephrine. They are characterized by episodes of hypertension, headache, palpitations, sweating and apprehension. See Hypertension.

Adrenocortical hyperplasia -- Increase in the number of cells of the adrenal cortex. Adrenal cortex secretes cortisol, androgens and aldosterone. Increased production of any or all of these hormones may result in a variety of disorders, such as Cushing's syndrome and hypertension. See Cushing's syndrome; hypertension.

Adrenocorticotropic hormone deficiency -- Not enough ACTH is produced by the pituitary gland. See ACTH.

Adrenoleukodystrophy -- Disturbance in brain substance caused by abnormal function of the adrenal gland.

Agglutination -- Clumping together.

Ahaptoglobulinemia -- Without haptoglobin in the blood. Condition is often seen with hemolytic anemia, severe liver disease and infectious mononucleosis. See Anemia, hemolytic; infectious mononucleosis.

Alcohol cardiomyopathy -- Disease of the myocardium (muscle layer) of the heart, due to chronic alcoholism. Results in enlargement of the heart. Heart muscle is weakened and cannot pump blood efficiently.

Alcoholic polymyopathy -- Disease affecting several muscles simultaneously. Caused by alcoholism. **Aldosteronism, primary** -- Overproduction of aldosterone, which is secreted by adrenal glands. Caused by adrenal hyperplasia (increase in number of adrenal cells) or a tumor of the adrenal gland (Conn's syndrome). Symptoms may include hypertension, muscle weakness or cramping, kidney disease and abnormal heart rhythm. See Adrenal hyperplasia; Conn's syndrome; hypertension.

Alkalosis, metabolic -- Abnormal condition in which body fluids are more alkaline than normal. Can result from loss of acid from prolonged vomiting or excess intake of bicarbonate.

Alkalosis, respiratory -- abdominal pain, diarrhea, appetite loss and brown skin. Abnormal condition when body fluids are more alkaline than normal. Caused by conditions that decrease the level of carbon dioxide in the blood, such as breathing too rapidly or congestive heart failure. See Congestive heart failure.

Alveolar edema -- Swelling of the smallest branches of the bronchial tubes (alveoli). **Ambiguous genitalia** -- External genitals that are not normal for the sex.

Amblyopias -- Reduced vision in an eye that appears to be normal when examined with an ophthalmoscope (an instrument used to examine the interior of the eye). Sometimes associated with strabismus. May also be caused by certain toxins.

Amenorrhea -- There are two categories of amenorrhea. In primary amenorrhea, menstruation has not begun in a young woman who has passed puberty and is at least 16 years old. Cause is usually unknown. Possible causes may include eating disorders, psychological disorders, endocrine disorders, congenital abnormality in which female organs are absent or abnormally formed, or participation in very strenuous athletic activities. In secondary amenorrhea, there is cessation of menstruation for at least 3 months in a woman who has previously menstruated. Causes include pregnancy, breast feeding, eating disorders, endocrine disorders, psychological disorders, menopause (usually 35 years of age or older), surgical removal of uterus or ovaries, or very strenuous athletic activities.

Amine -- Organic chemical compound containing nitrogen.

Amino acids -- Organic chemical compounds. They are the chief components of all proteins. The body contains at least 20 amino acids; 10 are ESSENTIAL. The body doesn't make or form these acids, so they must be acquired through diet.

Ampulla of Vater -- Enlarged area where the pancreatic duct and common bile duct come together before entering the %%duodenum (section of small intestine).

Amyloid -- Starchy substance.
Amyloid infiltration -- See Amyloidosis.
Amyloidosis -- Disease in which a waxy, starchlike, translucent material accumulates in tissues and organs, impairing function. Cause is unknown and is currently incurable. If kidneys are involved, kidney dialysis or a kidney transplant may be part of the treatment.
Amyotrophic lateral sclerosis (ALS; Lou Gehrig's disease) -- Progressive breakdown of spinal cord cells, resulting in gradual loss of muscle function. Not contagious or cancerous.
Anaphylaxis (Allergic shock) -- Severe, life-threatening allergic response to medications or other allergy-causing substances.
Androgenic arrhenoblastoma -- Ovarian tumor in which cells resemble those in male testes; they secrete male sex hormone. Causes appearance of male secondary sex characteristics in a woman, such as a husky, deep-pitched voice, excessive body hair and enlarged clitoris.
Andrenogenital syndrome -- Endocrine disorder resulting from adrenocortical hyperplasia. See Adrenal hyperplasia. Less than normal amounts of cortisol and greater than normal amounts of androgens are produced. This results in precocious puberty in boys and masculinization of the external genitals in girls. Usually a congenital disorder.
Anemia -- Condition in which the number of red blood cells or hemoglobin (oxygen carrying substance in blood) are inadequate.
Anemia, aplastic -- Serious disease characterized by decreased bone marrow production of all blood cells. Symptoms may include paleness, weakness, frequent infection, spontaneous bleeding from the nose, mouth, gums, vagina, rectum, brain and other sites, unexplained bruising, and ulcers in the mouth, throat or rectum. May be caused by disease in the bone marrow or destruction of the bone marrow by exposure to certain chemicals, anticancer drugs, immunosuppressive drugs or antibiotics. Cause is sometimes unknown. Curable if cause can be identified and treated successfully. If response to treatment is poor, complications of uncontrollable infections and bleeding may be fatal.
Anemia, autoimmune hemolytic -- Anemia due to the breakdown of an individual's blood cells by his own serum. Exact cause is unknown and still under investigation. See Serum.
Anemia, chronic hemolytic -- Anemia caused by an inherited disorder, such as hereditary spherocytosis, G-6-PD deficiency, sickle cell anemia or thalassemia. Currently no cure is known. See Anemia; hemolytic anemia; G-6-PD deficiency; sickle cell anemia; thalassemia.
Anemia, diserythropoietic -- Any anemia caused by a disorder that diminishes the body's normal ability to produce red blood cells.
Anemia, hemolytic -- Anemia due to the premature destruction of mature red blood cells. Bone marrow cannot produce red blood cells fast enough to compensate for those being destroyed.
Anemia, hypochromic -- Any of a large group of anemias characterized by a decreased concentration of hemoglobin in red blood cells. See Red cell indices.
Anemia, hypoplastic -- Anemia characterized by decreased bone marrow production of red blood cells.
Anemia, idiopathic acquired hemolytic -- Anemia characterized by a shortened lifespan of red blood cells. Cause is unknown, but it is not hereditary.
Anemia, iron deficiency -- Decreased number of circulating red blood cells or insufficient hemoglobin in the cells. Caused by inadequate supplies of iron.
Anemia, macrocytic -- Blood disorder characterized by abnormal presence of large, fragile red blood cells. Mean corpuscular hemoglobin (MCH) and mean corpuscular volume (MCV) are increased. See Red cell indices. Often the result of folic acid and vitamin-B12 deficiency.
Anemia, megalobastic (Folic acid deficiency) -- Anemia caused by folic acid deficiency. Often accompanied by iron deficiency anemia.
Anemia, microcytic -- Any anemia characterized by abnormally small red blood cells, usually associated with chronic blood loss or nutritional anemia, such as iron deficiency anemia. See Anemia, iron deficiency; anemia, megaloblastic; red cell indices.

Anemia, non-spherocytic hemolytic -- Inherited disorder of red blood cells in which shortened red cell survival is associated with membrane defects, unstable hemoglobins and intracellular defects. **Anemia, pernicious** -- Anemia caused by inadequate absorption of vitamin B12.
Anemia, pyridoxine-responsive -- Decreased red blood cells in circulation, which increase to normal with pyridoxine treatment.
Anemia, sickle cell -- Severe, incurable anemia that occurs in people who have an abnormal form of hemoglobin in their blood cells. It is an inherited disease.
Anemia, sickle cell trait -- See Sickle cell trait.
Anemia, sideroblastic--A special type of anemia in which the bone marrow deposits iron prematurely into red blood cells. These cells do not transport oxygen to the body as efficiently as normal cells. Anencephaly -- Absence of the brain.
Aneuploidy -- Any variation in chromosome number that involves individual chromosomes and not entire sets of chromosomes. There may be fewer chromosomes, as in Turner's syndrome, or more chromosomes, as in Down's syndrome. See Turner's syndrome; Down's syndrome. Abnormal traits vary depending on which set of chromosomes is involved.
Aneurysm -- Abnormal enlargement or ballooning of an artery. Caused by a weak artery wall.
Angina (Angina pectoris) -- Chest pain or pressure usually beneath the sternum (breastbone). Caused by inadequate blood supply to the heart. Often brought on by exercise, emotional upset or heavy meals in someone who has heart disease.
Angina pectoris -- See Angina.
Angiodysplasia -- Small blood vessel abnormalities.
Angioedema (Angioneurotic edema; hives) -- Allergic disorder characterized by skin changes with raised areas, redness and itching.
Angiomas -- Benign tumor made up of blood vessels or lymph vessels. Most are congenital.
Anion gap -- Measure combining laboratory analysis of sodium, chloride and bicarbonate. A quick, noninvasive calculation.
Ankylosing spondylitis -- Chronic, progressive disease of the joints, accompanied by inflammation and stiffness. Characterized by a BENT-FORWARD posture caused by stiffening of the spine and support structures. Cause is unknown but may be due to genetic changes or an autoimmune disorder. Currently considered incurable, although symptoms can be relieved or controlled. There have been cases of unexplained recovery.
Anorectal abscess -- Abscess occurring in the rectum (last segment of the large intestine) and anus (opening of the rectum on the body surface). See Abscess.
Anorexia -- Loss of appetite.
Anorexia nervosa -- Extremely complicated personality disorder, chiefly in young women, characterized by aversion to food, obsession with weight loss and various other symptoms. Anovulation-Failure of ovaries to produce, mature or release eggs. **Antibodies** -- Proteins created in blood and body tissue by the immune system to neutralize or destroy sources of disease.
Antigens -- Germs or other sources of disease that antibodies (produced by the immune system) neutralize or destroy. See Antibodies.
Anti-lipemic (Anti-lipidemic) -- Of or pertaining to a regimen, diet, agent or drug that reduces the amount of fat or fat-like substances (lipids) in the blood.
Antinuclear antibody (ANA) -- Substance that appears in the blood indicating presence of an autoimmune disease. See Autoimmune disease.
Aortic-valve stenosis -- Heart abnormality characterized by narrowing or stricture of the aortic valve due to a congenital malformation of the valve or fusing of segments of the valve, such as from rheumatic fever. See Rheumatic fever. This results in obstruction of blood flow out of the heart into the aorta; heart cannot pump effectively. Signs of the disease include intolerance for exercise, heart pain and heart murmur. Treatment usually includes surgery to repair the defective valve.
Aortoiliac occlusive disease -- Complete or partial blocking of the lower part of the aorta as it enters the leg, at the level of the groin.

Aplastic anemia -- See Anemia, aplastic.

Apnea -- Absence of spontaneous breathing.

Appendicitis -- Inflammation of the vermiform appendix (small tube that extends from the first part of the large intestine). Affects 1 in 500 people every year. Symptoms may include right lower abdominal pain, nausea, vomiting, constipation or diarrhea, and fever. Treatment includes prompt surgical removal of the appendix. Delay in surgery usually results in a ruptured appendix and peritonitis, which can be fatal. See Peritonitis.

Arachnoiditis -- Inflammation of the arachnoid membrane, a thin, delicate membrane enclosing the brain and spinal cord.

Arginosuccinic aciduria -- Presence of arginosuccinic acid in the urine. This is an inborn error of metabolism and causes mental retardation.

Arrhythmias -- Occasional or constant abnormalities in the rhythm of the heartbeat.

Arterial-occlusive disease -- Total or partial blockage of any large artery.

Arteriosclerosis -- Common disorder of the arteries characterized by thickening, loss of elasticity and calcification of artery walls. Results in decreased blood supply to the brain and lower extremities. Typical signs include pain on walking, poor circulation in feet and legs, headache, dizziness and memory defects. Condition often develops with aging or with nephrosclerosis, scleroderma, diabetes and hyperlipidemia. See Diabetes; nephrosclerosis; scleroderma.

Arteriovenous malfunction -- Problem at the junction of an artery and vein at the capillary level. **Arthritis** -- Inflammatory condition of the joints, characterized by pain and swelling. Also see Rheumatoid arthritis.

Ascites -- Accumulation of serous fluid in the abdominal cavity. It contains large amounts of protein and electrolytes. May be a complication of cirrhosis, congestive heart failure, nephrosis, cancer, peritonitis or various fungal and parasitic diseases. See Cirrhosis; congestive heart failure; nephrosis; cancer; peritonitis.

Asphyxia -- Loss of consciousness due to too little oxygen and too much carbon dioxide in the blood. If not corrected, it results in death.

Asthma -- Chronic disorder with recurrent attacks of wheezing and shortness of breath. **Astigmatism** -- Visual impairment caused by abnormal eye shape.

Astrocytomas -- Brain tumor composed of neuroglial cells (one of the two main kinds of cells that make up the nervous system). Usually grows slowly, but often a highly malignant tumor, called a glioblastoma, develops inside the astrocytoma. Complete surgical removal of an astrocytoma may be possible early in the development of the tumor, but not after it has invaded surrounding tissue.

Ataxia-telangiectasia -- Severe, hereditary, progressive disease beginning in early childhood. It results in lesion of a blood vessel formed by dilation of a group of small blood vessels (telangiectasias) of the eyes and skin, failure of muscles to coordinate (ataxia), including abnormal eye movements and immunodeficiency. This probably accounts for increased susceptibility to infections. Usually results in shortened life span.

Atopic dermatitis -- Chronic inflammatory disease of the skin; often associated with other allergic disorders that affect the respiratory system, such as asthma or hay fever. See Asthma. Cause is unknown, but may be an inherited or an immune system deficiency disease. Symptoms include itchy rash in skin creases, dry, thickened skin in affected areas, uncontrolled scratching and fatigue from loss of sleep due to intense itching. Flare-ups and remissions can occur throughout life. Treatment may relieve symptoms.

Atria -- Chamber allowing entrance into another structure. Usually refers to ATRIA of the heart, which allows transmission of blood into the larger chambers of the heart called the ventricles.

Atrial fibrillation -- Completely irregular heartbeat rhythm. In this case, it occurs in the top chambers of the heart. Sometimes it causes no symptoms. Sometimes the person may feel weak, dizzy or faint. Often, a normal heart rhythm can be restored with medication or an electric shock (electrocardioversion).

Atrophy -- Wasting away; diminishing in size such as a cell, tissue, organ or part. May result from disease, lack of use, aging or other influences.

Autoimmune -- Response directed against the body's own tissue.

Autoimmune disease -- Disease in which the immune system produces antibodies that attack the body's own tissues.

Autoimmune hemolytic anemia -- See Anemia, autoimmune hemolytic.

Autoimmune thyroid disease -- See Grave's disease.

B <u>INDEX</u>

Bacteremia -- Presence of bacterial germs in the bloodstream.

Bacterial endocarditis -- Noncontagious infection of the valves or lining of the heart.

Bacterial myocarditis -- Infection of the heart muscle caused by bacterial germs.

Baker's cyst -- Benign tumor on the back of the knee joint. Tumor consists of accumulated fluid that protrudes between two groups of muscles behind the knee. May result from injury or from diseases, such as arthritis or gout. See Arthritis; gout. Baker's cyst can be surgically removed if it becomes painful, unsightly or presses on blood vessels or nerves. If caused by disease, it usually disappears after successful treatment of the underlying disease.

Bartter's syndrome -- Inherited disease characterized by short stature, mental retardation, hyperaldosteronism and decreased potassium in the blood.

Benign -- 1) Tumor or growth that is neither cancerous nor located where it might impair normal function. 2) Harmless.

Bernard-Soulier syndrome -- Hereditary coagulation disorder marked by a mild decrease in the number of platelets circulating in the blood and abnormally shaped platelets. Following trauma and surgery, blood loss may be greater than normal; transfusion may be needed. The use of aspirin may provoke hemorrhage in people with this condition.

Beta-blockers -- Medications that reduce heart or blood vessel overactivity to improve blood circulation. Also used to prevent migraine headaches, hypertension and angina. See Hypertension; angina.

BILE SAND -- Thickened, gritty bile excreted by the liver into the gallbladder and bile ducts. Bile sand usually indicates the presence of infection of the gallbladder.

Biliary obstruction -- Blockage of the common or cystic bile duct, usually by one or more gallstones. Prevents normal bile flow into the small intestine.

Bilirubin -- Yellowish red blood cell waste product in bile the blood carries to the liver. It contributes to the yellow color of urine. Can cause jaundice if it builds up in the blood. Formed mainly by the breakdown of hemoglobin in red blood cells after the end of their normal life span.

Bilirubin, unconjugated -- Bilirubin that is insoluble in water. Bilirubin normally travels in the bloodstream to the liver, where it is converted to a water soluble (conjugated) form and excreted in the bile. Abnormally high levels of unconjugated bilirubin may be caused by liver damage, severe hemolytic anemia or Gilbert's disease. See Anemia, hemolytic; Gilbert's disease. Very high levels in a newborn require treatment with phototherapy or an exchange transfusion to prevent brain damage. Usually someone with a high unconjugated-bilirubin level appears jaundiced. See Jaundice.

Biopsy -- Removal of a small amount of tissue or fluid for laboratory examination; aids in diagnosis. **Bitemporal hemianopsic** -- Defective vision in which blindness occurs in the outer half of the visual field in each eye.

Blastic phase -- Immature stage of cell development.

Blastomycosis -- Infectious fungal disease that starts in the lungs. Occasionally it spreads through the bloodstream to other body parts, especially the skin. It is not contagious. Symptoms may include cough, chest pain, shortness of breath, chills, fever and drenching sweats. Usually occurs in the southeastern states and the Mississippi River Valley in the U.S. Fungus can cause severe, debilitating illness that may be fatal without treatment. With intensive treatment, it is usually curable in several weeks.

Blood -- Liquid pumped by the heart through arteries, veins and capillaries. It consists of a clear, yellow fluid called plasma and formed elements of cells. See Plasma. Blood's major function is to transport oxygen and nutrients to cells and remove from cells carbon dioxide and other waste products for detoxification and elimination.

Blood dyscrasias -- Condition caused by or relating to disease in which any component of the blood is abnormal or present in abnormal quantity.
Blood-factor deficiency -- Deficiency of one of the blood factors. See Factor I through Factor XIII. See Coagulation factors, page 855.
Bone disorders -- Any abnormality or disease of the bone or skeletal system.
Bone marrow -- Specialized soft tissue that fills the core of bones. Most of the body's red and white blood cells are produced in bone marrow.
Bone marrow disease -- Any disease affecting bone marrow. See Bone marrow.
Botulism -- Serious form of food poisoning caused by eating contaminated food containing a toxin that severely affects the nervous system. It is caused by a bacteria found in contaminated or incompletely cooked canned foods (especially home canned), undercooked sausage and smoked meats or fish. Symptoms develop suddenly 18 to 36 hours after eating contaminated food and include blurred vision, drooping eyelids, slurred speech, swallowing difficulty, vomiting, diarrhea and weakness of arms and legs that may lead to paralysis. Overall death rate is 10 to 25%. Outcome is usually good with prompt treatment.
Brain infarctions -- Localized area of brain tissue death resulting from lack of oxygen to that area because of an interruption in blood supply. Severity of symptoms following brain infarction depends on the location of the infarct and the extent of damage. See Infarction.
Bronchial tubes (Bronchi) -- Hollow air passageways that branch from the windpipe (trachea) into the lungs. They carry oxygen into the lungs and pass waste gases (mostly carbon dioxide) out of the body. **Bronchiectasis** -- Lung disease in which bronchial tubes become blocked and accumulate thick secretions. Frequently secondary infections occur. Not contagious unless associated with tuberculosis. See Tuberculosis. Symptoms may include cough, shortness of breath, malaise, fatigue and anemia. See Anemia. Treatment allows most people to lead nearly normal lives.
Bronchitis -- Acute or chronic inflammation of the bronchial tubes. Acute bronchitis is usually caused by a virus, although secondary bacterial infection is common. May also be caused from breathing chemical irritants (fumes, smoke, dust). Symptoms include cough, fever, chest discomfort and sometimes wheezing. Treatment includes rest, acetaminophen, expectorants to loosen mucus, increased fluid intake and antibiotics to fight bacterial infection.
Bronchodilator -- Any member of a group of drugs that dilates bronchial tubes and makes air passage in and out of the lungs easier. Help relax constricted tubes.
Bronchogenic carcinoma -- Malignant tissue growth in the lung, which may be caused by cigarette smoking, air pollution, metastasis from another cancer site or an unknown cause. Symptoms may include persistent cough, wheezing, chest pain, blood in the sputum, weakness, fatigue and weight loss. Only 25% of tumors may be removed surgically, however other treatment may help relieve symptoms. Survival rate after 5 years is less than 10%.
Brucellosis (Undulant fever) -- Illness caused by the brucella bacteria, which is transmitted to humans from animals. Characterized by fever, severe sweating, anxiety, generalized aching and abscesses in the bones, spleen, liver, kidney or brain. With treatment, it is rarely fatal, although complications can cause permanent disability.
B-Thalassemia -- Hemolytic anemia caused by decreased production of beta chains of hemoglobin in red blood cells. See Anemia, hemolytic; thalessemia.
C INDEX
Cachexia -- General poor health and malnutrition, including weakness and muscle wasting. Usually associated with serious disease.
Calcification -- Process by which calcium from the blood is deposited abnormally into tissues from injury, infection or aging. Often it is part of healing and not a sign of active disease.
Calcium -- Component of blood that helps regulate the heartbeat, transmit nerve impulses, contract muscles and form bone and teeth.
Calcium disorders -- Imbalance in the amount of calcium in the blood. Too much or too little can cause serious, sometimes life-threatening, medical problems.

Calculi -- Stones formed of mineral salts. Usually found within hollow organs or ducts. They can cause obstruction and inflammation. Kinds of calculi include gallstones and kidney stones. See Gallstones; kidney stones.

Cancer -- See Carcinoma.

Cannula -- Tube for insertion into a vessel or body cavity.

Capillary -- Smallest blood vessels in the body.

Capillary precipitation -- Settling of solid substances formerly in solution in the bloodstream.

Carcinoma -- Malignant tumor that tends to invade surrounding tissue; it may travel to distant regions of the body. Also see Cancer.

Cardiac distress -- Any condition causing difficulty in heart's normal functioning.

Cardiac glycosides -- Family of drugs used to treat heart disease. Digitalis is the outstanding cardiac glycoside.

Cardiac tamponade -- Compression of the heart due to collection of blood in the sac enclosing the heart (pericardium). Usually caused by a ruptured blood vessel in the heart muscle or by a penetrating wound. This is a life-threatening emergency requiring immediate medical treatment.

Cardiomyopathy (Hypertrophic cardiomyopathy) -- Disorder of the heart muscle usually associated with alcoholism, although there are some other causes. The heart muscle is weakened and cannot efficiently pump blood. May be curable if the underlying cause is curable. Some patients are candidates for a heart transplant.

Cardiorespiratory disease (Cardiopulmonary disease) -- Any disease affecting the heart and lungs.

Cardioversion -- Restoration of normal rhythm of the heart by electrical shock.

Casts -- Gelled protein particles on the walls of kidney tubules that break off and are washed out by urine. The presence of casts in urine is an abnormal finding caused by kidney disease.

Cataracts -- Clouding of the eye lens. A common cause of vision loss. Most commonly occurs in people over age 70. Congenital cataracts occur in newborns as genetic defects or from the mother having rubella (German measles) during the first 3 months of pregnancy. Other causes are rare. Usually curable with surgical removal of the lens. Special eyeglasses or contact lenses are needed after surgery.

Catheter -- Hollow tube used to introduce fluids into the body or to drain fluids from the body.

Cation-anion -- Positively charged ion attracted to the positive electrode in electrolysis.

Celiac disease (Nontropical sprue) -- Congenital disorder caused by an intolerance for gluten, a protein present in most grains. Gluten triggers an allergic reaction in the small intestine, which prevents the intestine from absorbing nutrients. Symptoms include poor appetite, abdominal bloating, fatigue and pale, bad-smelling stool that floats on water. Treatment includes a high protein, high calorie, gluten-free diet and vitamin-mineral supplements. Recovery is usually complete with treatment.

Cephalopelvic disproportion (CPD) -- Obstetric condition in which an infant's head is too large or the birth canal is too small to permit normal labor and delivery. A Cesarean operation is necessary to deliver the infant, unless the CPD is mild, then vaginal delivery may be possible.

Cervical spondylosis -- Degenerative changes of bones in the neck that place pressure on nerves and muscles to the arms, legs and bladder. May be caused by arthritis, injury or outgrowths of bone that may occur with aging. See Arthritis. Symptoms include pain in neck and shoulders, numbness and tingling in arms, hands and fingers, muscle weakness, dizziness, headache and double vision. Loss of bladder control and leg weakness may occur with advanced disease. Treatment usually relieves symptoms; rarely, surgery is required.

Cervix -- Lower third of the uterus, which protrudes into the vagina.

Charcot's disease (Neuropathic joint disease) -- Chronic, progressive degeneration of a joint, which is the result of an underlying neurological disorder. Characterized by swelling, heat, bleeding into the joint and instability of the joint. Early treatment may prevent further damage to the joint. Extensive disease may require amputation.

Chemical inhibition -- Process of retarding, arresting or restraining a chemical reaction.

Chemical profile (SMAC) -- Cost is about $24.00. This profile of tests is performed on an electronic machine and includes from 12 to 36 blood-chemistry determinations, including those listed in other profiles. See Profile.

Chemotherapy -- Treatment of cancer with medication that kills cancer cells without harming healthy tissue. Used to treat cancers that cannot be completely cured or treated with surgery or radiation. **Cholangitis** -- Infection or inflammation of the bile ducts (biliary tract) that drain bile from the gallbladder to the small intestine. Usually caused by gallstone formation and bile duct blockage. Symptoms include fever, belching, nausea, vomiting and pain in the upper right abdomen. Sometimes pain occurs in chest, upper back or right shoulder. Usually requires hospitalization. To prevent recurrences and possible complications, surgery to remove the gallbladder and stones is often performed after an acute attack. See Gallstones; kidney stones.

Cholecystitis -- Gallbladder inflammation usually caused by a gallstone that cannot pass through the cystic duct. See Gallstones.

Choledocholithiasis (Biliary calculus; biliary stone) -- Stone formed in the biliary tract. See Kidney stones. May lead to cholangitis if stone cannot pass spontaneously into small intestine. See Cholangitis. **Cholelithiasis (Gallstone)** -- Stones in the gallbladder that may or may not cause symptoms. If symptoms occur, surgery to remove the gallbladder is recommended to prevent complications of cholecystitis or cholangitis. See Cholecystitis; cholangitis; kidney stones; gallstones. Symptoms may include colicky pain in upper right abdomen or between shoulder blades, nausea, vomiting, belching or bloating, intolerance for fatty foods and jaundice. See Jaundice.

Cholestasis intrahepatic -- Interruption in the flow of bile to the biliary tract. May be caused by hepatitis, drug and alcohol use, pregnancy and metastatic liver cancer. See Hepatitis. **Chondromalacia** -- Abnormal softening of cartilage.

Chondromalacia patellae -- Occurs after knee injury. Characterized by swelling, pain and degenerative changes in the kneecap that are revealed by an X-ray examination.

Choriocarcinoma -- Malignancy arising in the uterus associated with pregnancy, abortion or hydatidiform mole. See Hydatidiform mole.

Christmas disease -- See Hemophilia.

Chromatin mass -- Portion of the cell nucleus that carries the genes of inheritance.

Chromophobe adenoma -- Tumor of the anterior portion of the pituitary gland; cells do not stain with acid or basic dyes. These tumors are usually not malignant and are associated with decreased function of the pituitary gland.

Chromosome -- Structures inside the nucleus of living cells that contain hereditary information. Defects in chromosomes cause many birth defects and inherited diseases.

Chronic -- Long-term; continuing. Chronic illnesses are usually not curable, but they can often be prevented from worsening. Symptoms usually can be controlled.

Chronic bronchitis -- Inflammation caused by repeated irritation or infection of the bronchial tubes. Causes them to thicken, narrow and lose elasticity. Symptoms include frequent cough, shortness of breath and sputum that is thick and difficult to cough up. Treatment includes stopping cigarette smoking and avoiding air pollution and other irritants, taking expectorants, bronchial drainage and deep breathing exercises. Sometimes medication is prescribed to dilate bronchial tubes.

Chyle -- Lymph and droplets of triglyceride fat in a stable emulsion. See Lymph. Lymph forms a milky fluid taken up by special structures in the intestinal tract during digestion of food.

Circle of Willis -- Network of blood vessels at the base of the brain, formed by the interconnection of several arteries that supply blood to the brain.

Cirrhosis -- Chronic scarring of the liver, leading to loss of normal liver function.

Citrullinuria -- Presence of large amounts of citrulline in the urine, plasma and cerebrospinal fluid. Citrulline is involved in producing urea.

Coagulation defects (Coagulopathy) -- Disruption of blood clotting mechanisms, resulting in hemorrhaging or internal bleeding. Complication of an underlying disorder.

Coagulation factors -- Chemical compounds necessary for blood to clot. See Factor I through Factor VIII.

Coccidioidomycosis (Valley fever) -- Infection caused by breathing spores of a fungus found in soil. It is not contagious. The disease is most common in desert areas of California, Arizona and Texas. Symptoms often resemble a common cold or influenza. See Influenza. Spontaneous recovery usually occurs in 3 to 6 weeks. Rarely, the infection can spread throughout the body and brain causing a life-threatening illness.

Cold agglutinins -- Antibodies that cause red blood cells to clump together at low temperatures. Mycoplasma pneumonia and infectious mononucleosis are two of several illnesses that cause a high number of cold agglutinins in the blood. See Infectious mononucleosis.

Colitis -- Inflammatory condition of the large intestine. It can occur in episodes, such as irritable bowel syndrome, or it can be one of the more serious, chronic, progressive, inflammatory bowel diseases, such as ulcerative colitis. See Ulcerative colitis. Irritable bowel syndrome is characterized by bouts of colicky abdominal pain, bloating, diarrhea or constipation, and fatigue, often due to emotional stress. Treatment includes stress reduction, diet changes and sometimes medication.

Collagen disease -- See Connective tissue disease.

Collagen-vascular disease -- See Connective tissue disease.

Collagen-vascular-autoimmune disease -- See Autoimmune disease. Examples of this disease are scleroderma and lupus erythematosus. See Scleroderma; lupus erythematosus, systemic.

Complement -- Series of enzymes in normal blood that interacts with antigens and antibodies.

Condyloma -- Wart-like growth on the mucous membrane or skin of the external genitals or around the anus.

Congenital -- Present at, and existing from, the time of birth.

Congenital anomalies -- Abnormality of the body present at birth; a birth defect. May be inherited or caused by conditions occurring while the fetus grows in the uterus.

Congenital hypothyroidism (Cretinism) -- Deficiency or lack of thyroid hormone secretion during fetal development. In infants it is characterized by breathing difficulties, jaundice and hoarse crying. See Jaundice. Infants diagnosed and treated before age 3 months usually grow and develop normally. If left untreated, child will suffer irreversible mental retardation, stunted growth and bone and muscle dystrophy. **Congestive heart failure** -- Complication of many serious diseases in which the heart loses its full pumping capacity. Blood backs up into other organs, especially the lungs and liver.

Conjunctivitis -- Inflammation of the lining of the eyelids and the covering of the white part of the eye. Caused by infection, allergy or chemical irritation. Usually lasts 2 to 3 weeks but can become a chronic condition.

Connective-tissue disease (Collagen disease) -- Any one of many abnormal conditions characterized by diffuse immunologic and inflammatory changes in small blood vessels and connective tissue. Some collagen diseases include systemic lupus erythematosus, scleroderma, polymyositis and rheumatic fever. See Lupus erythematosus, systemic; scleroderma; polymyositis; rheumatic fever.

Conn's syndrome -- Disorder of the adrenal cortex. See Adrenal cortex. Usually a noncancerous tumor that causes primary aldosteronism. See Aldosteronism, primary.

Coproporphyria -- See Porphyria.

Corneoscleral flaccidity -- Abnormal softness of the cornea and sclera of the eye.

Corneoscleral rigidity -- Abnormal inflexibility of the cornea and sclera of the eye.

Coronary artery bypass surgery -- Using a section of the patient's leg vein to bypass a partial or complete blockage in the coronary artery system. (Coronary arteries supply blood to the heart muscle.) Surgery may be performed to provide relief from angina pectoris, to restore blood to the heart muscle after myocardial infarction (heart attack) or to prevent a possible myocardial infarction (if the coronary arteries have narrowed or are blocked). Angina pectoris is cured in almost all cases. Probability of future heart attacks is reduced. See Angina pectoris; myocardial infarction.

Coronary artery disease -- Hardening and narrowing of the coronary arteries that provide blood to the heart muscle. The blood supply is decreased due to narrowing of the arteries; heart cells do not receive adequate oxygen. This disease often results in angina pectoris or myocardial infarction. Treatment can prolong life and improve its quality. Treatment may include medication, diet change, an exercise program and sometimes surgery. See Angina pectoris; myocardial infarction.

Coronary insufficiency -- Condition of the main arteries in the heart in which they supply an insufficient amount of oxygen to the cells of the heart. This is a serious increase in symptoms that, without intervention, may lead to myocardial infarction. Acute coronary insufficiency is also called unstable angina, preinfarction angina or intermediate syndrome. See Myocardial infarction.

Coronary occlusion -- Hardening and narrowing of one or more of the coronary arteries that provide blood supply to the heart. Narrowing is usually caused by atherosclerosis and sometimes spasms of the artery. When this occurs, adequate oxygen can no longer be provided to the heart muscle cells.

Coronary-risk profile -- Cost is about $40.00. Blood tests performed include Total Cholesterol, page 640, and Triglycerides, page 700. See Profile.

Craniopharyngiomas -- Congenital pituitary tumor appearing most often in children and adolescents. Characterized by increased pressure on the brain, vomiting, severe headaches, stunted growth, defective vision, change in behavior and infant-like genitals (in children). Development of the tumor after puberty results in cessation of menstruation in women and impotence and loss of sex drive in men.

Creatinine -- Substance formed from the metabolism of creatine, which is found in blood, urine and muscle tissue. Elevated creatinine in the blood usually indicates the presence of kidney disease. **Crepitus** -- Crunching sound similar to the sound made when tissue paper is crushed.

Cretinism -- Deficiency of thyroid hormone secretion during fetal development or early infancy. In children over age 2, it results from chronic autoimmune thyroiditis. Characterized by breathing difficulties, jaundice and hoarse crying in infants and stunted growth and mental deficiency in children. See Thyroiditis; jaundice. Without treatment, irreversible mental retardation occurs.

Crohn's disease (Regional enteritis) -- Inflammation of any part of the gastrointestinal tract that extends through all layers of the wall of the intestine. Symptoms include abdominal pain, cramping, diarrhea and sometimes fever and bloody stools. Complications include obstruction of the bowel, intestinal fistula, abscesses in the abdomen and around the rectum or anus, and bowel perforation (a hole in the wall of the intestine). May occur intermittently.

Cryoglobulins -- Abnormal blood proteins that separate from blood at low laboratory temperatures and redissolve when warmed. Cryoglobulins in blood are usually associated with immunologic disease. People with this condition may experience Raynaud's phenomenon if subjected to cold temperature. See Raynaud's phenomenon.

Crystal-induced arthritis -- Inflammation of a joint characterized by crystallization of fluids in a joint space.

Cushing's disease (Cushing's syndrome) -- Condition due to tumors of the adrenal cortex or the anterior lobe of the pituitary gland. More common in women. Symptoms include fatness of the face, neck and trunk, softening of the spine, absence of menstruation, dusky complexion with purple markings, hypertension, muscular weakness and other serious symptoms. See Hypertension.

Cushing's syndrome -- See Cushing's disease.

Cyst -- Sac or cavity filled with fluid or disease matter.

Cyanosis -- Bluish discoloration of skin, lips and nails. Caused by lack of oxygen.

Cystic fibrosis -- Inherited disease in which mucus-producing glands throughout the body, especially in the pancreas and lung, fail to produce normal enzymes and mucus.

Cystic tumors -- Tumors with cavities or sacs containing a semisolid or liquid material. **Cystinuria** -- Abnormal presence of cystine (an amino acid) in the urine. Also inherited defect in the kidney, characterized by excessive excretion of cystine and other amino acids in the urine. Can result in kidney or bladder stones. See Kidney stones.

Cytomegalovirus (CMV) infection -- Viral infection caused by cytomegalovirus. Characterized by weakness, fever, swollen lymph nodes, pneumonia and enlarged liver and enlarged spleen. See Pneumonia.

Cytotoxic -- Having a negative effect upon cells.

Cytotoxic agents -- Medications used to destroy cancerous cells with minimal harm to healthy cells.

D INDEX

DIC -- See Disseminated intravascular coagulation.

Delirium tremens (DTs) -- Acute, sometimes fatal, psychotic reaction caused by excessive intake of alcoholic beverages over a long period of time. Usually seen after withdrawal from heavy alcohol intake. Symptoms include mental confusion, excitement, hallucinations, anxiety, tremors of the tongue and extremities, fever, sweating and stomach and chest pain. An episode of DTs is considered a medical emergency.

Demyelinating disease -- Outer wrapping (myelin sheath) of the nerves or nerve fibers is destroyed. One example is multiple sclerosis. See Multiple sclerosis.

Dermatitis -- Inflammatory condition of the skin, characterized by redness and pain or itching. The type of skin rash or lesions that occur may suggest a particular allergy, disease or infection. The condition may be chronic or acute; treatment is specific to the cause.

Dermatofibromas -- Fibrous, tumorlike nodule of the skin most commonly found on the arms or legs. Requires no treatment. It is sometimes associated with systemic lupus erythematosus. See Lupus erythematosus, systemic.

Dermatomyositis -- Inflammation of connective tissue, with degenerative changes in muscles and skin. This causes weakness and muscle wasting, especially in the arms and legs. Cause is unknown.

Detached retina -- Separation or tear of the light-sensitive tissue at the back of the eye (retina) from the eye. Symptoms include light flashes or floating spots in the field of vision, blurred vision, partial loss of vision or gradual vision loss. Often curable with prompt surgical treatment.

Diabetes -- Any of various diseases characterized by an excessive discharge of urine.

Diabetes insipidus -- Disorder of the hormone system caused by a deficiency of antidiuretic hormone (ADH) normally secreted by the pituitary gland. Usually a temporary condition. Characterized by passage of large amounts of diluted, colorless urine (up to 15 quarts a day), unquenchable thirst, dry skin and constipation.

Diabetes mellitus: Insulin dependent -- Inability to produce enough insulin to process carbohydrates, fat and protein efficiently. Treatment requires insulin injections.

Diabetes mellitus: Non-insulin dependent -- Disease of metabolism characterized by the body's inability to produce enough insulin to process carbohydrates, fat and protein efficiently. Most prevalent among obese adults. Often controlled with weight loss, exercise and diet.

Diabetic acidosis -- See Diabetic ketoacidosis.

Diabetic ketoacidosis -- Serious complication of diabetes mellitus in which the body produces acids that cause fluid and electrolyte disorders, dehydration and sometimes coma.

Diabetic retinopathy -- Disorder of the innermost coat of the back of the eyeball. Seen most frequently in people who have had poorly controlled insulin dependent diabetes mellitus for several years. See Diabetes mellitus: insulin and noninsulin dependent. Characterized by microscopic dilation of capillary vessels, hemorrhages, exudates and the formation of new blood vessels.

Dialysis -- Process of separating crystals and other substances in a solution by the difference in their rate of diffusion through a semipermeable membrane.

Diaphoresis -- Profuse perspiration.

Diaphragm -- Large, thin muscle that separates the chest cavity from the abdominal cavity. **Diaphragmatic paralysis** -- Complete loss of function of the diaphragm. See Diaphragm. The diaphragm is used with each breath of air.

DiGeorge's syndrome -- Congenital disorder characterized by severe immunodeficiency, birth defects and absence of the thymus and parathyroid glands. Death usually occurs by age 2, often caused by infection.

Diphtheria -- Highly contagious infection, primarily affecting the mucous membranes of the nose, throat and larynx. May lead to difficulty breathing, airway obstruction and shock. The bacteria that causes diphtheria produces poisons that spread to the heart and central nervous system. Usually curable with prompt treatment. Delayed treatment may result in death or long-term heart disease.

Diploidy -- Having two full sets of chromosomes.

Disease -- Process representing a departure from normal health.

Diserythropoietic anemia -- See Anemia, diserythropoietic.

Disseminated intravascular coagulation -- Serious disruption of blood clotting mechanisms, resulting in hemorrhaging or internal bleeding. Condition is a complication of an underlying disorder.
Diverticula -- Small, pouch-like projections in the wall of the colon.
Diverticulitis -- Inflammation of diverticula. During periods of inflammation, person experiences crampy pain and fever. White blood cells increase to fight off infection.
Down's syndrome -- Condition associated with a chromosome abnormality, usually trisomy of chromosome 21. See Trisomy. Symptoms and findings include a small, flattened skull, short, flat-bridged nose, an abnormal fold at the inner edge of the eyes, short fingers and toes, and moderate to severe mental retardation.
Duchenne muscular dystrophy -- Abnormal congenital condition characterized by progressive weakness and wasting of the leg and pelvic muscles. Often involves the heart muscle. Affects only male children. Symptoms usually begin between the ages of 3 and 5. Currently not curable.
DUMPING SYNDROME -- Group of symptoms that is a complication of surgical removal of all or part of the stomach. Often experienced 1 to 6 months after surgery. It becomes a serious problem in 1 to 2% of all patients. Symptoms include weakness, faintness, decreased blood pressure, abdominal cramping, diarrhea, sweating and anxiety.
Duodenal lesions -- Abnormalities in the duodenum, such as ulcers, tumors or inflammatory reactions. **Duodenal ulcer** -- Peptic ulcer located in the duodenum, which is the first segment (about 10-inches long) of the small intestine that leads from the stomach. See Peptic ulcer.
Duodenitis -- Inflammation of mucous membrane lining of the duodenum. **Duodenum** -- First portion of the small intestine.
Dwarfism -- Underdevelopment of the body. **Dyspnea** -- Difficulty breathing.
Dysentery -- Inflammation of the intestine, especially the colon; may be caused by chemical irritants, bacteria, viruses, parasites or protoza. Characterized by frequent, bloody stools, abdominal pain and ineffective, painful straining to have a bowel movement (tenesmus).
Dysfibrinogenemia -- Congenital disorder in which fibrinogen is present in the blood, but does not function normally. See Fibrinogen.
Dysproteinemia -- Derangement of the protein content of the blood.
E INDEX
Eclampsia (Toxemia of pregnancy) -- Extremely serious disturbance in blood pressure, kidney function and the central nervous system, including seizure and coma. May occur from the 20th week of pregnancy until 7 days after delivery. Cause is unknown.
Ectopic ACTH production -- Adrenocorticotropic hormone production (ACTH) at some site other than the pituitary gland.
Ectopic pregnancy -- Pregnancy that develops outside the uterus. The most common site is one of the narrow tubes that connect each ovary to the uterus (Fallopian tube). Other sides include the ovary or abdominal cavity.
Edema -- Accumulation of fluid under the skin (swelling), in the lungs or elsewhere.
Electrolyte package -- Cost is about $20.00. Blood tests performed include Sodium, page 184, Potassium, page 178, Carbon Dioxide, page 692, and Chloride, page 114. See Profile.
Elliptocystosis -- Hereditary disorder in which red blood cells (erythrocytes) are oval in shape, instead of round, and have pale centers. Disorder may occur in a variety of anemias.
Embolism -- Sudden blockage of a blood vessel by an embolus. See Embolus.
Embolus -- Clot, foreign object, air, gas or a bit of tissue or fat that circulates in the bloodstream until it becomes lodged in a blood vessel.
Encephalitis -- Acute inflammation of the brain, usually caused by a contagious viral infection. May also be caused by lead poisoning, leukemia or as a vaccine reaction. See Leukemia. Symptoms in severe cases may include impairment of vision, speech and hearing, vomiting, headache, personality changes, seizures and coma. In mild cases, symptoms include fever and malaise. Death or complications, such as permanent brain damage, are most common in infants and people over 65. People in other age groups

usually recover completely.

Endobronchial -- Within the bronchial tubes.

Endocrine disorders -- Any disorder involving the endocrine system. The endocrine system is made up of organs that secrete hormones into the blood to regulate basic functions of cells and tissues. Endocrine organs are pituitary, thyroid, parathyroid, adrenal glands, pancreas, ovaries (in women) and testicles (in men).

Endometriosis -- Disorder in women in which tissue resembling inner lining of the uterus (endometrium) is found at unusual locations in the lower abdomen. Tissue may be found on the outside of the ovaries, behind the uterus, low in the pelvic cavity, on the intestinal wall and rarely, at other sites far away. **Enteritis** -- Inflammation of the mucous membrane lining of the small intestine.

Enterocolitis -- Inflammation of the mucous membrane lining of the small and large intestine.

Ependymomas -- Tumor in the brain or spinal cord that is usually benign and slow growing.

Epilepsy -- Disorder of brain function. There are several forms of epilepsy, each with its own characteristics. Cause is usually unknown (75% of the time) but may be due to brain damage at birth, severe head injury, drug or alcohol abuse, brain infection or brain tumor. It is incurable, except in rare cases where brain tumor or infection is treatable. Anti-seizure drugs can prevent most seizures and allow a nearly normal life.

Epilepsy, focal -- Small part of the body begins twitching uncontrollably. The twitching (seizure) spreads until it may involve the entire body. The person does not lose consciousness.

Epilepsy, grand mal -- Affects all ages. Person loses consciousness, stiffens, then twitches and jerks uncontrollably and may lose bladder control. Seizure may last several minutes and is often followed by a deep sleep or mental confusion.

Epilepsy, petit mal -- Affects children mostly. Child stops activity and stares blankly around for a minute or so and is unaware of what is happening.

Epilepsy, temporal lobe -- Person suddenly behaves out of character or inappropriately, such as becoming suddenly violent or angry, laughing for no reason or making bizarre body movements, including odd chewing movements.

Erythroblastosis fetalis (Rh-incompatibility) -- Incompatibility between an infant's blood type and that of its mother. Results in destruction of the infant's red blood cells (hemolytic anemia) after birth by antibodies from mother's blood. See Anemia, hemolytic. Treatment includes an exchange transfusion. **Erythropoiesis** -- Formation of red blood cells.

Erythropoietic porphyrias -- Inherited disorder in which there is an abnormal increase in the production of porphyrins (chemicals in all living things). Erythropoietic porphyria is characterized by production of large quantities of porphyrins in the blood-forming tissue of bone marrow. Symptoms include sensitivity to light, abdominal pain and neuropathy.

Erythropoietic protoporphyrias -- Disease characterized by itching, redness and edema after short exposure of the skin to sunlight.

Esophageal rings -- Muscular fibers that surround the esophagus.

Esophageal varices -- Enlarged veins on the lining of the esophagus subject to severe bleeding. They often appear in patients with severe liver disease. See Varices.

Esophagitis -- Inflammation of the mucous-membrane lining of the esophagus. May be caused by infection, irritation, or most commonly, from the backflow of stomach acid.

Esophagus -- Hollow tube that provides passage from the back of the throat to the stomach.

Essential hypertension -- See Hypertension.

Eunuchoidism -- Deficiency of male hormone, which results in abnormal tallness, small testes and deficient development of secondary sex characteristics, sex drive and potency.

Exchange transfusion -- Introduction of whole blood in exchange for 75 to 85% of an infant's circulating blood. Blood is repeatedly withdrawn in small amounts and replaced with equal amounts of donor blood. This procedure is performed in infants to treat erythroblastosis fetalis. See Erythroblastosis fetalis.

Exudate -- Matter that penetrates through vessel walls into adjoining tissue. Production of pus or serum.

Accumulation of fluid in a cavity.

F INDEX

FSP (Fibrin split products) -- Results from the breakdown of fibrinogen by plasmin (an enzyme). See Fibrin.

Factor I -- Fibrinogen needed for blood to clot.

Factor II -- Prothrombin needed for blood to clot.

Factor III -- Tissue thromboplastin needed for blood to clot. **Factor IV** -- Calcium needed for blood to clot.

Factor V -- Proaccelerin needed for blood to clot.

Factor VI -- Accelerin needed for blood to clot.

Factor VII -- Proconvertin needed for blood to clot.

Factor-VII deficiency -- Deficiency of normal clotting factor. Can be inherited or acquired. This deficiency commonly causes nosebleeds, easy bruising and bleeding gums.

Factor VIII -- Anti-hemophilic factor needed for blood to clot.

Factor IX -- Plasma thromboplastin component needed for blood to clot. **Factor X** -- Stuart factor (autoprothrombin C) needed for blood to clot. **Factor XI** -- Plasma thromboplastin antecedent needed for blood to clot. **Factor XII** -- Hageman factor needed for blood to clot.

Factor XIII -- Fibrin-stabilizing factor needed for blood to clot.

Familial hypoproteinemia -- Inherited abnormal decrease in the amount of protein in the blood.

Familial myoglobinuria -- Inherited condition in which myoglobin appears in urine. Causes include vigorous, prolonged exercise and severe injuries, such as a broken bone. See Myoglobin.

Familial xanthurenic aciduria -- Inherited deficiency disorder of xanthine oxidase that causes physical and mental retardation.

Fanconi's syndrome -- Rare, usually congenital disorder characterized by aplastic anemia, bone abnormalities, olive-brown skin pigmentation, abnormally small head, small gonads and kidney-function abnormalities. See Anemia, aplastic. Adults can get a form of the syndrome as a result of heavy-metal poisoning. It also may occur after a kidney transplant.

Fetal hypoxia -- Absence of sufficient oxygen to sustain life in a fetus. **Fibrillation** -- Quivering of heart muscle fibers.

Fibrin -- Protein formed from fibrinogen by the action of blood clotting.

Fibrin split products -- See FSP.

Fibrinogen -- Protein in the blood needed for blood clotting.

Fibrinolysis -- Breakdown of fibrin by enzyme action.

Fibrinolysis, secondary -- Process by which connective tissue is dissolved by the action of enzymes as a result of some disease process.

Fibrinolysis, systemic -- See Fibrinolytic disorders.

Fibrinolytic disorders -- Disease process characterized by dissolution of connective tissue by the action of enzymes.

Fibrocystic disease (Breast lumps) -- Disorder of the female breast characterized by nonmalignant lumps. Cause is unknown. Lumps may be accompanied by generalized breast pain, especially before menstrual periods. Lumps often enlarge before menstrual periods, then shrink afterward.

Fibroids -- Abnormal growth of cells in the muscular wall of the uterus (myometrium). Uterine fibroids are composed of abnormal muscle cells and are almost always benign. Cause is unknown. Usually decreases in size without treatment after menopause.

Fibromas -- Benign neoplasm of fibrous or fully developed connective tissue. **Fibrosis** -- Generation of fibrous tissue, such as in a scar.

Fibrous ankylosis -- Immobility and consolidation of a joint from disease caused by fibrous tissue. **Fibrous tissue** -- Tissue that is made up of fibers.

Filariasis -- Disease caused by the presence of parasitic worms or larvae in body tissue. Worms are round, long and threadlike. They are common in tropical and subtropical regions. They enter the body as microscopic larvae through the bite of a mosquito or other insect then infest the lymph glands and channels. Treatment is not very effective. After many years, this disease usually results in elephantiasis, characterized by tremendous swelling of the external genitals and legs. Overlying skin becomes dark, thick and coarse.

Fissures -- 1) Cleft or groove on the surface of an organ, often marking division of the organ into parts, as the fissures of the brain. 2) Crack-like lesion of skin.

Fistulas -- Abnormal passage between two organs or between an internal organ and the body surface. **Fluoresce** -- Emits light while exposed to light.

Focal epilepsy -- See Epilepsy, focal.

Focal seizures -- Convulsions brought about by a disease process or injury to an identifiable part of the brain. Such seizures usually affect only one side or a specific area of the body as opposed to a generalized seizure, which is likely to involve all muscle groups in the body.

Fulminating infection -- Infection that occurs suddenly, with great intensity.

G INDEX

G-6-PD (Glucose-6-phosphate dehydrogenase) -- Enzyme normally found in most body cells. Deficiency is inherited and makes red blood more prone to destruction.

Galactorrhea -- Breast milk flow not associated with childbirth or breast feeding. It may be a symptom of a pituitary gland tumor.

Galactosemia -- Inherited disease of infants in which milk cannot be digested. Milk should be eliminated from the infant's diet to prevent malnutrition, liver disease, kidney disease and mental retardation. **Gallbladder disease** -- Any disease involving the gallbladder or biliary tract. The gallbladder is a reservoir for bile; the biliary tract is the passageway that transports bile to the small intestine. Gallbladder disease is a common, often painful condition requiring surgery. It is commonly associated with gallstones and inflammation.

Gallstones -- Calculus or stone formed in the gallbladder. See Cholelithiasis.

Ganglioneuroblastoma -- Tumor of nerve cells.

Ganglioneuroma -- Benign tumor composed of nerve fibers.

Gangrene -- Dead tissue. Develops when a wound becomes infected or tissue is destroyed by an accident.

Gastrin -- Hormone that stimulates the production of gastric acid or stomach acid.

Gastrinoma -- Benign or malignant gastrin-secreting islet-cell tumor of the pancreas. There is an overproduction of gastric acid often resulting in an ulcer.

Gastritis -- Irritation, inflammation or infection of the stomach lining. Cause is sometimes unknown but may be due to excess stomach acid, food allergy, viral infection or adverse reaction to alcohol, caffeine or some drug. Symptoms may include nausea, diarrhea, abdominal pain, cramps, fever, weakness, belching, bloating and loss of appetite. Usually curable in 1 week, if cause is eliminated. **Gastroenteritis** -- Inflammation of the stomach and intestines accompanying many digestive-tract disorders. Causes may include bacterial, viral or parasitic infections, food poisoning, food allergy, excess alcohol consumption or emotional upset. Symptoms are the same as gastritis. See Gastritis. Recovery usually occurs within 1 week.

Gastrointestinal disease -- Any disorder of the gastrointestinal tract, which includes the mouth, esophagus, stomach, duodenum, small intestine, cecum, appendix, the ascending colon, transverse colon, descending colon, sigmoid colon, rectum and anus.

Gastrointestinal disorders -- Any condition or disease relating to any part of the digestive system, including the mouth, esophagus, stomach, small intestine, large intestine and rectum. May also include some conditions relating to the liver, gallbladder and pancreas.

Gastrointestinal (GI) symptoms -- Any symptoms relating to the stomach or intestine. Some common GI symptoms include vomiting, diarrhea, constipation, bloating and heartburn.

Gaucher's disease -- Rare familial disorder of fat metabolism characterized by an enlarged spleen, enlarged liver and abnormal bone growth in early childhood.

Genital herpes -- Viral infection of the genitals transmitted by intercourse or oral sex. Genital herpes may increase the risk of cervical cancer. Symptoms include painful blisters on the genitals that can cause painful urination, fever, malaise and enlarged lymph glands. Currently incurable, but treatment can relieve symptoms.

Germ cell tumors -- One of three types of cancer of the ovary. Arises in the ovum (egg). Prognosis is often poor because tumors tend to progress rapidly. Advances in chemotherapy may improve outcome. Rarely may occur in children.

Gigantism -- Condition in which the body or a body part grows excessively, sometimes due to an overactive pituitary gland.

Gilbert's disease (Gilbert's syndrome) -- Benign hereditary condition characterized by jaundice and high bilirubin levels in the blood. See Jaundice. No treatment is required.

Glanzmann's thrombosthemia -- Rare, inherited hemorrhagic disease. See Hemorrhagic disease. Platelet cells cannot cluster normally; clots do not form and hemorrhage occurs. Transfusion with platelets is usually effective in stopping any bleeding.

Glaucoma -- Abnormally increased pressure within the eyeball that may produce severe, permanent vision defects. It is the most preventable cause of blindness. If diagnosed and treated early, it rarely results in permanent loss of vision.

Globulins -- Class of proteins that are insoluble in water but soluble in saline solutions. **Glomerular** -- Of or pertaining to a glomerulus.

Glomerulonephritis (Post-infectious, acute or chronic) -- Inflammation of glomerulus. See Glomerulus. Damaged glomeruli cannot effectively filter waste products from the blood. Acute glomerulonephritis may follow streptococcal infection of the throat or skin. Kidney symptoms usually begin 2 to 3 weeks after strep infection.

Glomerulus -- Tiny structure composed of blood vessels. One of several structures that make up a nephron in the kidney. See Nephron. There are about 1.25-million nephrons in each kidney that filter the blood and remove wastes.

Glucagonoma -- Glucagon-secreting tumor of the islet cells of the pancreas. Glucagon increases blood sugar.

Glucocortocoid deficiency -- Decreased amount of hormone from the adrenal gland that increases production of glycogen.

Glycogen -- Substance formed from glucose, stored chiefly in the liver. When the blood-sugar level is too low, glycogen is converted back to glucose for the body to use as energy.

Glycogen-storage disease (Glycogenosis) -- Any of a group of inherited disorders of glycogen metabolism. An enzyme deficiency causes glycogen to accumulate in abnormally large amounts in the body.

Goiter -- Enlargement of the thyroid gland, which causes a swelling in the front part of the neck. **Gonadal** -- Pertaining to gonads.

Gonadal impairment -- Decreased function of the gonads. See Gonads. Testes in men; ovaries in women.

Gonadotropin -- Any hormone having a stimulating effect on the gonads.

Gonads -- Parts of the reproductive system that produce and release eggs (ovaries in the female) or sperm (testes in the male).

Gonorrhea -- Infectious disease of the reproductive organs and other body structures that is sexually transmitted (venereal disease). The most prominent symptom is a thick, green-yellow discharge from the penis or vagina. Antibiotics usually effect a cure.

Gout -- Recurrent attacks of joint inflammation caused by deposits of uric acid crystals in the joints. It can be very painful.

Grand mal epilepsy -- See Epilepsy, grand mal.

Granulocytic leukemia -- See Leukemia, granulocytic.

Granulomas -- Nodule of firm tissue formed as a reaction to chronic inflammation, such as from foreign bodies or bacteria.

Granulomatosis -- Formation of multiple granulomas. Each has nodules of granulated tissue forming a

tumorlike mass.
Granulomatosus colitis -- See Crohn's disease.
Graves' disease -- Disorder of the thyroid gland occurring most often in women. Characterized by bulging eyes, rapid pulse rate, profuse sweating, restlessness, irritability and weight loss.
Growth hormone deficiency -- Deficiency of hormone that results in dwarfism.
Guillain-Barre syndrome -- See Polyneuritis.

H INDEX

HDL -- High density liproprotein.
Hageman factor (Factor XII) -- Deficiency of this factor results in prolonged bleeding. See Factor XII.
Hand-Schueller-Christian disease -- Group of three symptoms that may occur in any of several disorders. Symptoms include marked protrusion of eyeballs (exophthalmos), diabetes insipidus and bone destruction. See Diabetes insipidus.
Hartnup disease -- Hereditary disease that causes skin rash, unsteady gait and excess amino acids in the urine.
Hashimoto's thyroiditis -- One of several kinds of thyroid gland inflammation. **Heart attack** -- See Myocardial infarction.
Heinz bodies -- Granular deposits in red blood cells from precipitation of proteins. They are present in certain hemolytic anemias. See Anemia, hemolytic.
Hemangioma -- Benign tumor made up of a mass of blood vessels.
Hematoma -- Collection of blood that has escaped from a blood vessel and is localized in an organ or tissue.
Hematuria -- Abnormal presence of blood in the urine. May be gross (can actually see the blood) or microscopic (seen only under a microscope). Is usually a sign of kidney disease or urinary tract disorder. **Hemochromatosis** -- Disease in which excessive iron accumulates in the liver, pancreas and skin, resulting in liver disease, diabetes mellitus and a bronze skin color. See Diabetes mellitus: insulin and noninsulin dependent.
Hemoconcentration -- Decrease of the fluid content of the blood, with resulting increase in concentration of blood cells.
Hemodilution -- Increase in fluid content of blood, with resulting decrease in concentration of blood cells.
Hemoglobin-C disease -- Inherited blood disorder characterized by a moderate, chronic hemolytic anemia and associated with the presence of hemoglobin C, an abnormal form of the red cell pigment. See Anemia, hemolytic.
Hemoglobin-C trait -- Relatively common abnormal hemoglobin in which lysine replaces glutamic acid in the hemoglobin molecule.
Hemolysis -- Process by which red blood cells breakdown and hemoglobin is released. Occurs normally at the end of the life span of a red blood cell. It may also occur abnormally with certain diseases or conditions such as hemolytic anemia. See Anemia, hemolytic.
Hemolytic -- Condition in which red blood cells break down and release the hemoglobin they contain. One example is hemolytic anemia. See Anemia, hemolytic.
Hemolytic anemia -- See Anemia, hemolytic.
Hemolytic disease -- Disorder characterized by the premature destruction of red blood cells. May or may not result in anemia, depending on the ability of the bone marrow to increase production of red blood cells.
Hemolytic episode -- Separation of hemoglobin from red blood cells.
Hemolytic jaundice -- Jaundice caused by severe hemolytic anemia, which results in high levels of unconjugated bilirubin. Leads to a jaundiced appearance. See Bilirubin, unconjugated; anemia, hemolytic; jaundice.
Hemophilia -- Inherited deficiency of a blood clotting factor that may result in bleeding episodes. Characterized by bleeding into joints, muscles and skin, excessive bleeding from minor cuts, nosebleeds

and blood in urine.

Hemophilus influenzae (haemophilus influenza, Type-B) -- Bacteria that causes numerous diseases in children. Two of these diseases are especially serious. Meningitis (infection of the brain and spinal cord) can cause death or permanent brain damage. Epiglottitis is a condition of the throat in which the child can choke to death.

Hemoptysis -- Coughing up blood from the respiratory tract. Blood-streaked sputum can occur with minor upper respiratory tract infections. A greater amount of blood may indicate a serious disease or infection.

Hemorrhagic disease -- Medical problem accompanied by uncontrolled bleeding. Hemorrhagic disease of the newborn is rare because it is customary to give vitamin K to the mother just before delivery or to the infant immediately after birth.

Hemorrhagic gastritis -- Inflammation of stomach accompanied by bleeding from stomach lining. **Hemorrhoids** -- Dilated (varicose) veins of the rectum or anus. Usually caused by straining during bowel movements, although pressure from a rectal tumor or pregnancy may cause them. Symptoms may include rectal bleeding, pain, itching or mucus discharge after bowel movements and a lump that can be felt in the anus. If hemorrhoids are very large, there may be a sensation that the rectum has not emptied completely after a bowel movement.

Heparin therapy -- Course of treatment with medication that prolongs blood clotting time. Used to prevent or treat blood clots.

Heparinized -- To render blood non-clottable with heparin. For example, tubes used to collect blood often have heparin in them so blood does not coagulate.

Hepatic -- Of or affecting the liver.

Hepatic coma -- Stupor or coma caused by waste products in the blood that are toxic to the brain. Normally, waste products are neutralized by the liver, but due to extensive liver damage they continue to circulate in the blood. Can cause death.

Hepatic disease -- Any disease involving the liver, including many types of hepatitis and cirrhosis. **Hepatic dysfunction** -- Poor liver function.

Hepatitis -- Inflammatory liver condition characterized by jaundice, enlarged liver, loss of appetite, abdominal discomfort, abnormal liver function, dark urine and clay-colored stool. See Jaundice. Can be caused by bacterial or viral infection, parasites, alcohol, drugs or blood transfusions with incompatible blood. Symptoms may be mild, severe or life-threatening.

Hepatitis-B -- Form of viral hepatitis caused by the hepatitis-B virus. Characterized by rapid onset of acute signs and symptoms. See Hepatitis. Usually enters the body through blood transfusions contaminated with the virus or by the use of contaminated needles or instruments. Infection may be very severe and result in prolonged illness, cirrhosis or death. See Cirrhosis.

Hepatitis profile -- Cost is about $18.00. Blood tests performed include hepatitis-B surface antigen, antibody to core antigen and antibody (IgM) to A virus. These are all covered under Antibody Screening Test, page 52. See Profile.

Hepatocellular injury -- Injury of liver cells.

Hepatomas (Malignant liver tumor; hepatocellular carcinoma) -- Malignant tumor that begins in the liver (primary site of cancer), as opposed to liver cancer that has spread from another site. **Hepatotoxicity** -- Tendency of a substance, usually a medication or alcohol, to have a destructive effect on the liver.

Hereditary -- Transmitted genetically from generation to generation. **Hereditary anti-edema** -- Inherited condition that prevents accumulation of fluid.

Hereditary spherocytosis -- Inherited disorder characterized by small, spherical red blood cells, leading to anemia because abnormal cells are fragile. See Anemia.

Hernia -- Protrusion of an internal organ through a weakness or abnormal opening in the muscle around it. The most common types are inguinal hernia (in groin), femoral hernia (in groin), incisional hernia (at surgery site), umbilical hernia (at navel) and hiatal hernia. See Hiatal hernia. Umbilical hernias rarely require surgery. Other hernias are usually curable with surgery.

Herpes -- Herpes type-1 causes common cold sores, which appear around the mouth. Herpes type-2 (HSV-2) is a viral infection of the genitals transmitted by sexual intercourse. Type-2 herpes infection can be transmitted to a newborn from an actively infected mother. It can be fatal to the child.

Hgb-C disease (Hemoglobin-C disease) -- See Hemoglobin-C trait.

Hiatal hernia -- Abnormal weakness or opening in the diaphragm. Allows a portion of the stomach to protrude through the diaphragm. If symptoms occur (often there are none), they usually appear at least 1 hour after eating and may include heartburn, belching and sometimes difficulty swallowing. Treatment usually relieves symptoms. Surgery is rarely required.

High-purine diet -- Diet of foods that are high in purines, including anchovies and sardines, organ meats, legumes and poultry. See Purine. Increased intake of purines may lead to development of uric acid stones (a type of kidney stone). See Kidney stones.

Histidinemia -- Hereditary defect of metabolism marked by excess histidine (an amino acid) in the blood and urine. Many people with this defect show mild mental retardation and improper speech development.

Histology -- Science dealing with the microscopic identification of cells and tissue. **Histoplasmosis** -- Fungal infection from breathing dust that contains fungus spores or through direct contact into an open skin wound. Fungus is found in the feces of birds and bats and in soil contaminated by feces. In the U.S., disease is most prevalent in the Mississippi and Ohio River Valleys. Although the acute disease is benign, other forms are very serious and may be fatal. Usually curable with 3 months of treatment using antifungal drugs.

Hodgkin's disease -- Malignant tumor of the lymph glands characterized by progressive enlargement of the lymph nodes, loss of appetite, weight loss, fever, itching skin, night sweats and anemia. See Anemia. **Hodgkin's lymphoma** -- See Hodgkin's disease.

Homocystinuria -- Rare, hereditary defect of metabolism, marked by excess homocystine (an amino acid) in the blood and urine. Many people with this disorder are mentally retarded and have bone disorders, cardiovascular disorders and an enlarged liver.

Humoral -- Relating to any fluid or semifluid of the body.

Huntington's chorea -- Rare, abnormal, hereditary condition characterized by involuntary, purposeless, rapid movements of various body parts, as well as progressive mental deterioration. Symptoms often appear in the 40s with death occurring about 15 years later.

Hydatidiform mole -- Disease occurring during early pregnancy resulting in death of the fetus and an overgrowth of tissue within the uterus.

Hydrocephalus -- Condition characterized by an excessive accumulation of fluid with the cranial vault. **Hydronephrosis** -- Caused by an obstruction in the tube that carries urine from the kidney to the bladder (ureter). Because urine cannot flow past the obstruction, it backs up into the kidney causing distention or dilation. Prolonged hydronephrosis eventually results in loss of kidney function; surgery to remove the obstruction may be necessary.

Hyper -- Abnormally increased; excessive.

Hyperalimentation -- Supplying total nutritional needs of patients who are unable to eat normally by intravenous feeding or by tube through the nose into the stomach. Provides nutrients containing essential proteins, fats, carbohydrates and vitamins.

Hypercalcemia -- Presence of excessive calcium in the blood. May result from tumor of the parathyroid gland (due to overproduction of parathyroid hormone), Paget's disease, some cancers, multiple fractures or prolonged immobility. See Paget's disease. May also occur from excessive ingestion of calcium, such as overuse of antacids that contain calcium.

Hyperchloremia -- Presence of excessive amounts of chloride in the blood. May result from severe dehydration, complete shutdown of kidneys and primary aldosteronism. See Aldosteronism, primary. **Hyperfibrinogenemia** -- Presence of excessive fibrinogen in the blood. See Fibrinogen. May indicate cancer of the stomach, breast or kidney or an inflammatory disorder.

Hyperfunctioning tumor -- Any tumor that leads to higher than normal action of the chemicals (usually hormones) usually secreted by the tissue from which the tumor arises. For example, hyperfunctioning tumor of the thyroid gland leads to an increase in thyroid hormone released. **Hyperinsulinism** -- Excessive secretion of insulin.

Hyperkalemia -- Abnormally high blood potassium level. May be seen in people who have suffered severe burns, crushing injuries, diabetic ketoacidosis or myocardial infarction. See Myocardial infarction. Also seen in those who have Addison's disease or kidney failure. See Addison's disease. **Hyperlipoprotenemia** -- Condition in which excessive lipoproteins (cholesterol and other fatty materials) accumulate in the blood.

Hypermagnesemia -- Elevated levels of magnesium in the blood. Most commonly occurs in people with kidney failure. Can also result from Addison's disease. See Addison's disease.

Hypernatremia -- Excess of sodium in the blood, usually caused by excessive loss of water and electrolytes. Symptoms include mental confusion, seizures and eventually coma.

Hyperoxaluria -- Hereditary defect of metabolism, marked by excessive oxalate in the urine. May result in kidney stones, early onset of kidney failure (due to calcium deposits in the filtering system) and calcium-oxalate deposits in other areas of the body.

Hyperparathyroidism -- Excessive amounts of parathyroid hormone circulating in the blood. Excess amounts increase blood levels of calcium (hypercalcemia) and decrease blood levels of phosphorus (hypophosphatemia).

Hyperphosphatemia -- Abnormally high level of phosphates in the blood. May result from bone diseases, healing fractures, hypoparathyroidism, diabetic acidosis or kidney failure. See Hypoparathyroidism; diabetic ketoacidosis.

Hyperploidy -- Condition of having one or more chromosomes in excess of the normal number. The result is unbalanced sets of chromosomes. One example of hyperploidy is Down's syndrome. See Down's syndrome.

Hyperprolinemia, Type-A -- Disorder of amino acid metabolism.

Hypertension (High blood pressure) -- Increase in the force of blood against the arteries as blood circulates through them. Often has no symptoms. Essential or primary hypertension, the most common kind, has no single identifiable cause. Secondary hypertension is caused by an underlying disease.

Hyperthyroidism -- Overactivity of the thyroid, an endocrine gland that regulates all body functions. **Hypertonic** -- Solution that contains substances that flow outward through a semipermeable membrane into a solution of lower concentration.

Hypertrophic anal papilla -- Excessive growth of the papilla of the rectum. See Papilla.

Hypertrophic cardiomyopathy -- See Cardiomyopathy.

Hypertrophy -- Increase in the size of a cell or group of cells. Causes an increase in the size of an organ or part.

Hyperventilation -- Breathing so rapidly that carbon dioxide levels in the blood are decreased, upsetting normal blood chemistry. Can be caused by fever, heart disease, lung disease or severe injury. Can also be caused by anxiety. May be accompanied by numbness and tingling of mouth, hands and feet, weakness and faintness.

Hypo -- Deficient; beneath; under.

Hypoalbuminemia -- Abnormally low levels of albumin (protein) in the blood.

Hypoalderostonism -- Deficiency of aldosterone secreted by the outer layer of the adrenal glands. May result from Addison's disease, salt-losing syndrome and toxemia of pregnancy. See Addison's disease; salt-losing syndrome; toxemia; eclampsia.

Hypocalcemia -- Abnormally low level of calcium in the blood. May result from hypoparathyroidism or malabsorption of calcium. See Hypoparathyroidism. May be associated with Cushing's syndrome, kidney failure, pancreatitis or peritonitis. See Cushing's syndrome; pancreatitis; peritonitis.

Hypochloremia -- Abnormally low levels of chloride in the blood. Low chloride levels can occur from prolonged vomiting, intestinal fistula, chronic kidney failure and Addison's disease. See Addison's disease;fistulas.

Hypochromic anemia -- See Anemia, hypochromic.

Hypofibrinogenemia -- Abnormally decreased level of fibrinogen in the blood. See Fibrinogen. May result from disseminated intravascular coagulation, fibrinolysis, severe liver disease and some cancers. **Hypofunctioning tumor** -- Tumor that causes the anatomical part it encroaches on to have less than normal function.

Hypogammaglobulinemia -- Abnormally low levels of gammaglobulins in the blood, which results in an immunity deficiency. This makes you more susceptible to infectious diseases. You can be born with this condition or it can result from other diseases, such as nephrosis. See Nephrosis.

Hypoglycemia -- Abnormally low blood sugar level caused by abnormal function, not disease, of the pancreas. Excessive insulin produces symptoms of sweating, nervousness, weakness, nausea and rapid heartbeat. Excessive insulin may be caused by a tumor, called an insulinoma, that secretes too much insulin. Or it may result from a diabetic person injecting too much insulin. See Insulinoma. May also result from kidney failure, liver disease, alcoholism or decreased food intake. The brain must have glucose available at all times or brain cells are damaged. Hypoglycemia must be treated promptly. **Hypoglycemic syndrome** -- Condition caused by low blood sugar, characterized by cold sweat, low body temperature, headache, confusion, hallucinations and ultimately (if left untreated) convulsions, coma and death.

Hypogonadism -- Decreased functional activity of gonads, with hindered growth and slowed sexual development.

Hypogonadotropism -- Abnormal condition caused by decreased production of gonadotropins. See Gonadotropins.

Hypokalemia -- Below normal level of potassium in the blood. May result from aldosteronism, Cushing's syndrome, excessive loss of body fluids and licorice addiction. See Aldosteronism; Cushing's syndrome.

Hypolipoproteinemia -- Abnormally low levels of lipoproteins in blood.

Hyponatremia -- Less than normal concentration of sodium in the blood. Caused by excessive water in circulating blood or excessive loss of sodium from severe vomiting or diarrhea, or inadequate intake of sodium.

Hypooxaluria -- Decreased amount of oxalic acid in the urine.

Hypoparathyroidism -- Decreased production of hormones by the parathyroid glands, causing low calcium blood level.

Hypophosphatasia -- Inborn error of metabolism that causes difficulty building and healing bones. **Hypophysectomy** -- Surgical removal of the pituitary gland.

Hypopituitarism -- Underactivity of the pituitary gland, resulting in inadequate hormone production. **Hypoplasia** -- Incomplete development or underdevelopment of an organ or tissue, usually from a decrease in the number of cells.

Hypoplastic anemia -- See Anemia, hypoplastic.

Hypotension -- Abnormally low blood pressure. One symptom of shock.

Hypothyroidism -- Underactive thyroid gland, which results in decreased metabolic rate. Early symptoms may include decreased tolerance for cold, fatigue, unexplained weight gain, constipation and forgetfulness. If left untreated, the disorder may progress to myxedema and eventually coma. See Myxedema. Treatment includes thyroid replacement hormones.

Hypothyroidism, primary -- Caused by dysfunction of the thyroid gland and may be due to surgical removal of the thyroid, radioactive iodine treatment, Hashimoto's thyroiditis or inflammatory conditions, such as sarcoidosis. See Hashimoto's thyroiditis; sarcoidosis.

Hypothyroidism, secondary -- Caused outside the thyroid. It may result from decreased activity of the pituitary gland, which secretes thyroid stimulating hormone (TSH), dysfunction of the hypothalamus, which regulates TSH production, iodine deficiency in the diet or use of drugs that depress thyroid function.

I <u>INDEX</u>

Ichthyosis -- Skin condition in which skin is dry, thickened and fissured, resembling fish scales. Usually appears at or shortly after birth; it may be associated with one of several rare syndromes. Treatment with bath oil or vitamin-A solution (retinoic acid) applied to the skin may help some types.

Ichythosis follicularis -- Skin disorder characterized by dryness, roughness and scaliness. **Idiopathic** -- Without known cause.
Idiopathic-acquired hemolytic anemia -- See Anemia, idiopathic-acquired hemolytic.
Idiopathic cold-agglutinin diseases -- Disease of unknown cause associated with laboratory findings of an agglutinin that acts only at relatively low temperatures.
Idiopathic hypertrophic subaortic stenosis (IHSS) -- Chronic heart condition that produces an enlarged heart muscle, which restricts the amount of blood the heart pumps. Condition may be inherited, but cause is usually unknown. Symptoms may include chest pain, shortness of breath, fainting, heart rhythm irregularity, heart murmur, swollen feet and ankles, and enlarged, tender liver. Usually curable with medication or surgery.
Idiopathic thrombocytopenic purpura (ITP) -- Bleeding into the skin and other organs due to a deficiency of platelets.
Ileitis -- See Crohn's disease.
Immune -- Resistance or protection against infection by the body's natural defenses. A person may be immune to one kind of infection but not immune to another. Some infections, such as measles or chickenpox, cause permanent immunity to that infection.
Immunodeficiency diseases -- Defects in the body's immune system. A healthy immune system protects the body against germs (bacteria, viruses, fungi), cancer (partial protection) and any foreign material that enters the body. When the system fails, the body becomes susceptible to infection and cancer. Can range from minor to very severe.
Immunoglobin-deficiency disease -- Illness caused by deficiency of a protein molecule with known antibody activity.
Immunomedicated disease -- Illness caused by medicines that decrease the efficiency of the immune system in preventing or decreasing severity of disease.
Immunosuppressive therapy -- Drugs used to prevent the body from forming a normal immune response. Therapy is used to treat diseases (especially when organs must be transplanted) when certain antibodies must be inactivated.
Immunotherapy -- See Immunosuppressive therapy.
Infarction -- Tissue death due to the obstruction of blood to that tissue.
Infectious mononucleosis -- Infectious viral disease that affects the liver, respiratory system and lymphatic system.
Inferior vena cava -- Large vein that returns unoxygenated blood to the heart from parts of the body below the midchest.
Inflammatory bowel disease -- Characterized by fever, pain, abscess formation, severe diarrhea, bleeding and ulceration of the intestine's mucous membrane lining. Cause is unknown. Treatment includes fluids, cortisone drugs, antibiotics, diet change and sometimes surgery.
Influenza -- Common, contagious respiratory infection caused by a virus. Incubation after exposure is 24 to 48 hours.
Insulinoma -- Benign (nonmalignant) tumor of insulin secreting cells of the islets of Langerhans in the pancreas. It results in excessive insulin production and is one of the main causes of hypoglycemia. See Hypoglycemia. It is a rare disease and very difficult to diagnose because symptoms are often vague and mimic neurologic and psychiatric disorders. Treatment is usually surgical removal of the tumor. Frequent high carbohydrate meals or medication may also be used.
Insulin-resistant states -- Severe insulin dependent diabetes mellitus that no longer responds to treatment with insulin. See Diabetes mellitus: insulin and noninsulin dependent.
Intermittent positive-pressure-breathing therapy -- Form of treatment for disorders of the lungs using a sophisticated, expensive instrument that forces air into the lungs by controlled positive pressure. Treatment is usually given by a trained pulmonary therapist or technician.
Interstitial -- Occupies space between tissues, such as interstitial fluid.
Interstitial fibrosis -- Formation of fibrous tissue between normal tissues.
Intestinal fistula -- Abnormal opening leading from the intestinal tract to another abdominal organ or to

the skin.

Intraepithelial neoplasia -- Small tumor or cancer in the epithelial layer of the skin.
Intravenously (I.V.) -- Through a vein.
Intrinsic factor levels -- Substance secreted by the stomach lining that is necessary for vitamin B-12 to be absorbed by the intestine. A deficiency of intrinsic factor results in pernicious anemia. See Anemia, pernicious.
Iodine-deficient goiter -- Enlarged thyroid gland due to too little iodine in the diet. Iodine is an essential trace element and is usually found in drinking water. Using small amounts of iodized table salt (if you live in an area with insufficient iodine in drinking water) prevents the occurrence of a goiter. A goiter causes a pronounced swelling in the front part of he neck. See Goiter.
Iritis -- Inflammation of tissues that support the iris (the ring of colored tissue around the pupil of the eye). Symptoms include eye pain, sensitivity to light and blurred vision. May be caused by infection that spreads to the eye from other body parts, injury to the eye or an autoimmune reaction. Often cause is unknown.
Iron-deficiency anemia -- See Anemia, iron deficiency.
Iron overload -- Too much iron in blood, liver or other organs.
Ischemia -- Decreased blood supply to a body organ or part.
Ischemic -- Condition in which there is decreased blood flow to a body organ or part.
Ischemic bowel disease -- Intestinal problems caused by inadequate supply of blood to the cells of the intestines.
Isichromosome -- Abnormal chromosome characterized by abnormal splitting of a chromosome during the process of duplicating itself. May cause inherited diseases or disorders.
Isoenzyme -- One of many forms of a protein catalyst differing in characteristics (chemical, physical, immunological) but catalyzing the same reaction. For example, lactate dehydrogenase may exist in five different forms.
Isothermal infusion -- Injection with a fluid at the same temperature as the recipient. **I.V.** -- See Intravenously.

J INDEX

Jaeger card -- Card with printed letters of varying sizes. Used to test vision.
Jaundice -- Condition of yellow skin, yellow whites of the eyes, dark urine and light-colored stools. It is a symptom of diseases of the liver and blood caused by abnormally elevated amounts of bilirubin in the blood.

K INDEX

Karotyping -- Determining the chromosome constitution of the nucleus of a cell. Useful in predicting abnormalities in a fetus before birth, using amniotic fluid to study cells.
Keloids (Cheloids) -- Overgrowth of scar tissue at the site of a wound on the skin. New scar tissue is elevated, rounded, firm and irregularly shaped. Occurs most often in young women and blacks. Sometimes requires local treatment or surgery.
Keratosis -- Any horny growth, such as a wart.
Keratosis follicularis -- Uncommon hereditary skin disorder characterized by small, horny growths that grow together to form brown or black, crusted, wart-like patches. They can spread rapidly, ulcerate and become covered with pus. Treatment includes large doses of vitamin-A by mouth, vitamin-A acid cream applied to lesions and sometimes steroids taken by mouth or applied to the skin.
Ketoacidosis -- Serious disorder that results from a deficiency or inadequate use of carbohydrates. Characterized by fluid and electrolyte disorders, dehydration and mental confusion. If left untreated, coma and death may occur. It is usually a complication of diabetes mellitus but may also be seen in starvation and rarely in pregnancy if diet is inadequate. See Diabetes mellitus: insulin and non-insulin dependent.
Ketone bodies -- Substances formed when the body rapidly breaks down fats to use for energy.
Ketonuria -- Presence of ketone bodies in the urine. Usually seen in people with uncontrolled diabetes mellitus or as a result of starvation. See Diabetes mellitus: insulin and non-insulin dependent.

Kidney shut down (Kidney failure; renal failure) -- Sudden failure of kidneys to function. Usually has a short, relatively severe course but is often curable.
Kidney stones -- Hard, unyielding material produced by the kidney. May lodge in the kidney or pass through the ureter, the bladder and finally the urethra to the outside of the body.
Klippel-Feil syndrome (Congenital short-neck syndrome) -- Rare, congenital malformation of the neck due to fewer than normal vertebrae in the neck or because vertebrae are joined together. Results in limited neck movement and a low hairline. May require no treatment. It can cause pressure on nerves; if this occurs, traction or surgery may be necessary.
Kyphosis -- Abnormal condition in which the upper spinal column (between the neck and midback) curves outward excessively. Sometimes occurs in adolescents. Usually causes no symptoms and requires no treatment. Can be caused by rickets or tuberculosis of the spine. See Rickets; tuberculosis. If very severe, may be treated with a back brace; rarely surgery is needed.

L INDEX

LDL -- Low density lipoprotein.
L/S ratio -- Ratio of lecithin to sphingomyelin. Abnormalities may represent the possibility of an immature or premature fetus.
Lactic acidosis -- Increased acidity in body due to accumulation of excessive lactic acid production.
Laennec's cirrhosis -- Cirrhosis of the liver associated with alcohol abuse. See Cirrhosis.
Laryngospasm -- Spasmotic closure of the larynx or voice box. When spasms occur, air cannot pass through the larynx properly. May occur with croup in infants, in tetany, caused by abnormally low calcium level in the blood, or in tetanus (lockjaw). Can be life-threatening if condition is severe. **Larynx** -- Part of the air passage connecting the throat with the trachea or windpipe.
Lateral sclerosis -- Degeneration of the lateral columns of the spinal cord.
Leprosy -- Chronic disease characterized by the production of fibrous connective-tissue lesions (granulomatous) of the skin, mucous membranes and peripheral nervous system (excluding the brain and spinal cord). It is not very contagious and requires prolonged, intimate contact to be transmitted to another person. The more serious form of leprosy may cause blindness and severe disfigurement. Treatment can result in improvement of skin lesions, but recovery of nerve damage is limited.
Lesion -- Injury or damage to an organ or tissue.
Leukemia, acute -- Malignant overgrowth of white blood cells in bone marrow or tissues that are part of the lymphatic system (lymph glands, spleen, liver). These excess cells accumulate and spill into the blood, eventually involving other tissues. Most common form of cancer in children.
Leukemia, granulocytic -- Malignant blood disease of granulocytes, a form of white blood cell.
Leukemia, lymphatic -- Cancer that primarily involves lymphatic cells. Affects children and adults. **Leukemia, lymphocytic** -- Very slow-growing cancer of blood-forming organs in older people. About 35% of all leukemia victims have this form of the disease. It is often discovered in a routine blood test for unrelated purposes.
Leukemia, monocytic -- Malignancy of blood-forming tissues in which the predominant cells are monocytes (a type of white blood cell). The disease has an erratic course characterized by malaise, fatigue, fever, weight loss, enlarged spleen, bleeding gums, anemia and unresponsiveness to therapy. See Anemia.
Leukemia, myeloblastic -- Malignancy of blood cells in which the predominant cells are myeloblasts (a form of white blood cell).
Leukemia, myelogenous -- See Leukemia, myelocytic.
Leukemia, myeloid -- Malignancy of white blood cells with polymorphonuclear cells predominant. **Leukemia, myelomonocytic** -- Malignancy of blood cells in which the predominant cells are monocytes and myelocytes.
Leukemia, myleocytic -- Disorder characterized by the unregulated, excessive production of myelocytes. See Myelocytes.
Leukoagglutinins -- Antibodies directed against white blood cells.
Liothyronine (T3 3) toxicosis -- Overactive thyroid function due to T3 poisoning.

Liver profile -- Cost is about $20.00. Blood tests performed include Bilirubin, Protein, LDL, Alkaline Phosphatase, SGOT, SGPT, Albumin, and Globulin. See Profile.
Lordosis -- Forward curvature of the lumbar spine (the small of the back).
Lumbar stenosis -- Narrowing or stricture in the lower part of the back.
Lupus erythematosus, systemic -- Inflammatory disease of connective tissue. Symptoms may include arthritis, swelling of the face and legs, anemia, mental changes, shortness of breath, hair loss and chest pain. See Arthritis; anemia. Treatment usually requires immunosuppressive steroid and non-steroid antiinflammatory drugs. It is not inherited or cancerous. Currently considered incurable.
Luteinization -- Process by which a follicle in the ovary transforms into a luteum. **Luteinized granulosa** -- Thick, scarred, yellow lesion.
Luteum -- Yellow-colored cyst.
Lymph -- Transparent, slightly yellow liquid found in lymph vessels throughout the body. Derived from tissue fluids.
Lymphatic -- Pertaining to lymph system of the body.
Lymphatic leukemia -- See Leukemia, lymphatic.
Lymphatic system -- Vast, complex network of vessels, valves, ducts, nodes and organs that help protect and maintain the internal fluid environment of the body. Responsible for transporting fats, proteins and other substances to the bloodstream. Lymph glands produce antibodies that help fight infections.
Lymphoblastic lymphoma (Lymphoblastoma; lymphoblastic lymphosarcoma) -- Malignant tumor of lymph tissue. Lymphomas are classified according to the predominant cell type causing the disease. Lymphoblastic lymphoma's predominant cell is structured similarly to the lymphoblast. Treatment for lymphoma includes intensive radiotherapy and chemotherapy.
Lymphocyte -- One of several types of white blood cell that help fight infection. **Lymphocytic leukemia** -- See Leukemia, lymphocytic.
Lymphocytic proliferative disease -- Disease with an overproduction of lymphocytes, one form of white blood cells.
Lymphoma -- Disorders involving new, abnormal growth or tumor of lymph tissue. Usually malignant but may be benign. Usually afflicts men.
Lymphoreticular malignancy -- Cancer of the reticuloendothelial cells of lymph nodes. See Reticuloendothelial system.
Lymphosarcoma -- Malignant tumor of the lymph glands. More common than Hodgkin's disease. See Hodgkin's disease.
Lysis -- Destruction or breakdown, as of a cell or other substance.
M INDEX
Macroamylaemia -- Excess of starch in the blood. **Macrocytic anemia** -- See Anemia, macrocytic. **Macroglobulinemia** -- See Waldenstrom's macroglobulinemia. **Macular disease** -- Stain, spot or thickening of the cornea.
Malabsorption syndromes -- Poor absorption of nutrients from the intestinal tract into the blood. **Malaise** -- Vague feeling of body discomfort.
Malaria -- Infection caused by a single cell parasite transmitted by the bite of an anopheles mosquito. Uncommon in the U.S., but often affects travelers or military personnel stationed in foreign countries. **Male menopause** -- Symptoms, such as depression, change in libido, impotence, in men at midlife. Many authorities claim no such condition exists.
Malignant -- Capable of causing destruction of normal tissue; may lead to death. Usually refers to cancer growth.
Mallory-Weiss syndrome -- Condition characterized by massive bleeding following a tear in the mucous membrane at the junction of the esophagus and stomach. Tear is usually caused from prolonged vomiting, most common in alcoholics or people who have an obstruction preventing food from passing out of the stomach into the small intestine. Surgery is usually required to stop bleeding.
Maple-syrup urine disease -- Hereditary defect of metabolism. Usually diagnosed in infancy because

it is recognized by the characteristic maple-syrup odor of urine. Other symptoms may include mental and physical retardation and feeding difficulties.

Mast cells -- Part of connective tissue.

Mastocytosis -- Overproduction of mast cells. May rarely infiltrate liver, spleen, bones, the gastrointestinal system and skin. May precede mast cell leukemia, which is a malignant disorder.

Mean corpuscular hemoglobin (MCH) -- See Red cell indices.

Mean corpuscular hemoglobin concentration (MCHC) -- See Red cell indices.

Meconium -- Thick, sticky, dark-green material that collects in the intestines of a fetus and forms the first stools of a newborn.

Meconium ileus -- Obstruction of the small intestine in the newborn caused by a plug of meconium. See Meconium. Often the plug may be dislodged by giving enemas. Rarely, surgery is required. Condition may be an indication of cystic fibrosis. See Cystic fibrosis.

Mediastinitis -- Inflammation of the mediastinum. See Mediastinum.

Mediastinum -- Central portion of the chest cavity that contains the heart and its large blood vessels, trachea (windpipe), esophagus, thymus gland and other structures and tissues. It separates the two lungs. It does not include the lungs.

Medulla -- Most internal part of a structure or organ. **Medullary** -- See Medulla.

Megaloblastic anemia -- See Anemia, megaloblastic.

Melanin -- Dark pigment of the skin, hair and iris of the eye. **Melanocytes** -- Cells that produce melanin.

Melanoma -- Any of a group of malignant tumors, primarily of the skin, made up of melanocytes. See Melanocytes. Most develop from a pigmented mole over a period of several months or years. **Meningioma** -- Hard, usually vascular tumor of the membranes covering the brain and spinal cord. Usually grows slowly. May invade the skull causing bone erosion and pressure on brain tissues. Usually occurs in adults, in some cases following head injury.

Meninges -- Thin membranes that cover the brain and spinal cord.

Meningitis -- Inflammation or infection of the meninges. See Meninges. It is contagious and may be caused by viruses, fungi or bacteria. Symptoms may include fever, headache, stiff neck, irritability, sensitivity of eyes to light, confusion, drowsiness or unconsciousness. Death or permanent brain damage may occur if treatment is delayed (especially in bacterial meningitis). Usually full recovery may be expected in 2 to 3 weeks, if there are no complications.

Meningocele (Meningoencephalocele) -- Hernia protrusion of the brain and its coverings through a defect in the skull.

Menke's kinky-hair syndrome -- Inherited disorder caused by a defect in intestinal absorption of copper. Characterized by the growth of sparse, kinky hair. Infants with syndrome suffer brain damage, retarded growth and early death.

Menopause -- Permanent cessation of menstruation. Occurs as early as age 35 or as late as age 55; usually spans 1 to 2 years. Menopause is only one event in the CLI-MACTERIC, a biological change in body tissue and body systems that occurs in both sexes between the mid-40s and mid-60s. **Menstrual** -- Pertaining to menstruation. See Menstruating.

Menstruating -- Normal discharge of blood and tissues through the vagina that come from the uterine lining. Lining builds up each month in preparation for a fertilized egg. If fertilization does not occur, lining is shed. This process is controlled by hormones and usually occurs about every 4 to 6 weeks.

Mesenteric adenitis -- Lymph glands in mesentery become inflamed. Symptoms may mimic appendicitis, but the pain is usually more generalized and does not become more severe. **Mesentery** -- Membranous folds that hold and suspend the small intestines.

Metabolic alkalosis -- Too much base in the body due to loss of acid.

Metabolism -- Sum of all the chemical and physical processes by which living substance is produced and maintained. Also includes the concept of the transformation by body cells by which energy is made available.

Metabolites -- Any substance produced by metabolism. See Metabolism.

Metachromatic leukodystrophy -- Inherited condition that causes blindness, mental retardation, rigidity and convulsions.

Metamorphopsia -- Defective vision in which objects appear distorted. Sometimes results from disease of the retina.

Metastasis -- Process by which cancerous cells or infectious germs spread from their original location to other parts of the body.

Metastatic -- Pertaining to metastasis. See Metastasis.

Metastatic cancer -- Cancerous cells that spread from their original location to other parts of the body. **Metastatic disease** -- Disease that has transferred from an organ or body part not directly connected to a new location, due to transfer of the germ. For example, tuberculosis is usually found in the lungs but can spread to bones and other organs. In this case, the lungs are the primary site of disease, and the bones or other organs are the site(s) of metastatic disease. See Tuberculosis.

Microaneurysms -- Microscopic aneurysms, characteristic of certain diseases. Capillary microaneurysms are often seen in the retina of the eye in diabetic retinopathy. See Aneurysms; diabetic retinopathy.

Microbes -- Microorganism (small, living organism) capable of producing disease. **Microcytic anemia** -- See Anemia, microcytic.

Miliary tuberculosis -- Acute infection associated with the spread of tuberculosis throughout the body through the bloodstream. Tiny tubercles (small, rounded masses produced by infection with mycobacterium tuberculosis, the germ causing tuberculosis) are formed in a number of organs. If treatment is not delayed, the infection can usually be successfully treated with a combination of medications. See Tuberculosis.

Mitogen -- Substance that triggers mitosis. See Mitosis.

Mitosis -- Type of cell division in which the body produces new cells for growth and repair of injured tissues.

Mitral regurgitation -- Defective closure of the heart's mitral valve, which allows some of the blood to backflow or regurgitate. Normally, the mitral valve allows blood to flow from the top left chamber of the heart (atrium) to the bottom left chamber of the heart (ventricle), but prevents blood from flowing back into the left atrium. Although there are several causes, rheumatic heart disease is the single most common cause of this condition. Symptoms include fatigue and slight breathlessness. Eventually the condition may progress and result in severe congestion of lungs. Surgery to replace or repair the mitral valve is required in patients with severe symptoms.

Mitral stenosis -- Calcification and decreased function of the heart's mitral valves.

Mitral valve -- Valves located in the heart between the left atrium and left ventricle.

Mitral valve prolapse -- Condition in which the mitral valve becomes FLOPPY, resulting in mitral regurgitation. See Mitral regurgitation.

Mixed connective tissue disease (MCTD) -- Disease affecting the entire body characterized by the combined symptoms of various collagen diseases. Symptoms may include joint pain, inflammation of muscles, non-deforming arthritis and swollen hands. May also affect esophagus and lungs. Treatment often includes administration of corticosteroids.

Monocytic leukemia -- See Leukemia, monocytic.

Mononucleosis -- See Infectious mononucleosis.

Monosomy -- Chromosomal abnormality characterized by the absence of one chromosome from the normally occurring pair of chromosomes. One example is Turner's syndrome. See Turner's syndrome. **Motility disorders** -- Any disorder or disease characterized by inability to remove intestinal waste contents efficiently.

Mucocele -- Dilation of a cavity with accumulated mucus secretion.

Mucopolysaccharides -- Chemicals that contain hexosamine combined with proteins.

Mucopolysaccharidosis -- Any of a group of genetic disorders caused by a defect in metabolism of mucopolysaccharides. Characterized by skeletal changes, mental retardation, clouding of the cornea and excessive mucopolysaccharides in urine. Currently there is no successful treatment.

Multinodular goiter -- Enlarged thyroid gland causing a swelling in the front part of the neck. See Goiter. Swelling is very irregular (multinodular). Rarely toxic or malignant; may occur with chronic inflammatory thyroid disease.

Multiple myeloma (Primary bone marrow cancer) -- Malignancy beginning in the plasma cells of the bone marrow. Plasma cells normally produce antibodies to help destroy germs and protect against infection. With myeloma, this function becomes impaired, and the body cannot deal effectively with infection.

Multiple sclerosis (MS) -- Chronic disorder affecting many nervous system functions. Patches of white matter in the brain and spinal cord break down and cannot conduct normal nerve impulses. Usually begins in young adulthood. Early signs of the disease are often vague, including visual problems, abnormal skin sensations and muscle weakness or imbalance. Later, symptoms may include marked weakness, speech difficulty, loss of bladder or bowel control, and extreme mood swings. Currently not curable. Symptoms can be relieved or controlled with treatment. One-third of MS patients have a mild, nonprogressive disease. Another third worsen slowly. The rest worsen rapidly.

Mumps -- Mild, contagious, viral disease that causes painful swelling of the salivary glands. Other symptoms may include fever, headache and sore throat. Rarely, other organs may become involved, including testicles, ovaries, pancreas, breasts or brain.

Muscular dystrophy -- Gradual deterioration of the muscles of the body, leading to increasing difficulty walking and moving.

Myasthenia gravis -- Disorder of muscles, especially the face and head, with increasing fatigue and weakness as muscles are used.

Mycoplasma pneumonia -- Lung infection caused by germ mycoplasma. **Myeloblastic leukemia** -- See Leukemia, myeloblastic.

Myelocele -- Saclike protrusion of the spinal cord through a congenital defect in the spinal column. **Myelocytes** -- Immature white blood cells normally found in bone marrow.

Myelogenous leukemia -- See Leukemia, myelocytic. **Myeloid leukemia** -- See Leukemia, myeloid. **Myelomonocytic leukemia** -- See Leukemia, myelomonocytic. **Myelocytic leukemia** -- See Leukemia, myelocytic.

Myelosuppressive -- Inhibiting bone marrow activity, resulting in the decreased production of blood cells and platelets.

Myocardial failure -- Condition that exists when the heart is no longer able to pump all the blood efficiently.

Myocardial fibrosis -- Formation of fibrous material in the heart.

Myocardial infarction (Heart attack) -- Death of heart muscle cells from reduced or obstructed blood flow through the coronary arteries.

Myocarditis -- Inflammation of the heart muscle (myocardium) that usually occurs as a complication of underlying illness, hypersensitive immune reactions, injury or radiation therapy. Symptoms may include fatigue, shortness of breath, irregular heartbeat and fever. Usually curable with detection and treatment of the underlying cause.

Myocarditis bacterial -- Inflammation of heart muscle (myocardium) caused by bacterial infection. **Myocardium** -- Heart muscle.

Myoglobin -- Chemical stored in muscle that contains iron and oxygen.

Myxedema -- Condition of swollen lips, thickened nose, swelling of the skin and mental dullness caused by reduced function of the thyroid gland. See Hypoparathyroidism.

N [INDEX]

Necrosis -- Localized death of tissue that occurs in groups of cells in response to disease or injury. **Neisseria meningitides** -- Bacteria that is often the cause of meningitis. See Meningitis. **Neoplasms** -- Any abnormal growth of new tissue.

Neoplastic diseases -- Disease characterized by abnormal growth of new tissue. Cell multiplication is uncontrolled and progressive. Can be benign or malignant.

Nephritis -- Any one of a large group of diseases of the kidney characterized by inflammation and abnormal function. One example of nephritis is glomerulonephritis. See Glomerulonephritis. **Nephron** -- Anatomical and functional unit of the kidney consisting of tubules and blood vessels. **Nephrosclerosis (Nephroangiosclerosis)** -- Involves small arteries and kidney's filtering system. Caused by hypertension. See Hypertension. If the condition is severe and left untreated, kidney failure and heart failure result.

Nephrosis (Nephrotic syndrome) -- Form of chronic kidney disease beginning in early childhood. Characterized by protein in the urine, swelling of skin and organs, and low protein and high cholesterol blood levels.

Nephrostomy tube -- Flexible plastic tube passed into an opening made in the kidney that leads outside the body.

Nephrotic syndrome -- See Nephrosis.

Neurinoma -- Tumor of the nerve covering. Usually benign, but may undergo malignant change. **Neuritis** -- Inflammation of a nerve. Can cause pain, numbness, paralysis or sensitivity of the affected area.

Neuroblastoma -- Highly malignant tumor that usually originates in the adrenal glands of young children. Tumor metastasizes early and widely to lymph nodes, liver, lung and bone. Prior to metastasis, treatment is often successful.

Neurofibroma -- Fibrous tumor of nerve tissue.

Neurogenic -- 1) Forming nervous tissue or stimulating nervous energy. 2) Originating in the nervous system.

Non-Hodgkin's lymphoma (Lymphosarcoma) -- Malignant tumor of the lymph glands, which is more common than Hodgkin's disease. See Hodgkin's disease. Cause is unknown, but viral infection may be a factor. Symptoms may include swollen, rubbery, non-tender lymph glands anywhere in the body, weight loss, malaise, anemia, jaundice and bleeding from the digestive tract. See Anemia; jaundice. Usually curable with radiation therapy and anticancer drugs. The potential for cure varies according to the cell type discovered from biopsy of the lymph nodes.

Non-specific liver disease -- Poor liver function in the absence of a known cause.

Non-spherocytic hemolytic anemia -- See Anemia, non-spherocytic hemolytic.

Nystagmus -- Involuntary, rapid movements of the eyeball. Usually caused by an underlying disease.

O [INDEX](#)

Obstructive jaundice (Cholestasis) -- Interruption in the flow of bile through any part of the biliary tract. Causes can occur in or outside the liver. Causes outside the liver may be a gallstone, tumor in the common bile duct or cancer of the pancreas. For causes within the liver, see Intrahepatic cholestasis.

Occlusion -- Closing or obstruction. Usually describes a blockage in blood vessels.

Occult -- Hidden from view; difficult to observe directly.

Opacified -- Impervious to light rays or X-rays.

Optic atrophy -- Degeneration of the optic nerve.

Optic neuritis -- Inflammation of the nerve that conducts vision impulses from the eye to the brain. **Osteoarthritis (Degenerative joint disease)** -- Degeneration of cartilage at a joint and growth of bone SPURS that inflame surrounding tissue. Can be caused by stress on the joint due to activity and aging or from an injury to the joint lining. Symptoms include stiffness and pain of the affected joint. Cold, damp weather often increases pain.

Osteochondritis dissecans -- Inflammation of bone and cartilage, which results in pieces of cartilage splitting off into the affected joint.

Osteochondromas -- Benign tumors made of bone and cartilage.

Osteochondromatosis -- Occurrence of multiple osteochondromas. See Osteochondromas.

Osteomalacia -- Abnormal condition resulting in softening of bone. Accompanied by weakness, fracture, pain and weight loss. May be caused by a diet lacking in phosphorus, calcium or vitamin D, lack of exposure to sunlight or malabsorption.

Osteomyelitis -- Infection of the bone and bone marrow caused by bacteria, usually staphylococcus. Bacteria are usually introduced directly by trauma or surgery, but may travel through the bloodstream from an infected organ or tissue, such as from a middle ear infection or pneumonia. See Pneumonia. Usually curable with prompt, aggressive treatment. Requires hospitalization for observation and administration of intravenous antibiotics.

Osteoporosis -- Loss of normal bone density, mass and strength, leading to increased porousness and vulnerability to fracture. Usually occurs in women after menopause. Treatment includes a well-balanced, nourishing diet, specific vitamin-mineral supplements, exercise and sometimes estrogen replacement. Treatment can halt, and may reverse, bone deterioration.

Ovarian agenesis -- Congenital absence of ovaries resulting in sterility. **Overhydration** -- Too much fluid in tissues.

P INDEX

Paget's disease (Osteitis deformans) -- Gradual, progressive bone disease, characterized by bones breaking down and regenerating excessively. New bone is fragile and weak. It is not cancerous. **Pancreatic disease** -- Any disease of the pancreas.

Pancreatitis -- Inflammation of the pancreas. Chronic pancreatitis usually follows recurrent attacks of acute pancreatitis. Pancreas gradually becomes unable to supply digestive juices and hormones necessary for good health.

Panhypopituitarism -- Complex syndrome marked by deficiency of hormones secreted by the pituitary gland. It is very rare. Most often caused by a tumor of the pituitary gland. In children, it results in dwarfism and is characterized by dysfunction of metabolism, sexual immaturity and growth retardation. **Papilla** -- Small nipple-like projection or elevation.

Papilledema -- Swelling of the optic disk caused by increased intracranial pressure. Sometimes seen with serious conditions, such as a brain tumor, hemorrhage in the brain or swelling of the brain after head trauma.

Papilloma -- Benign tumor of the skin.

Paranasal-sinus disease -- Any disease or disorder of one of the sinuses in the skull adjacent to the nose structure. There are eight paranasal sinuses.

Parapatellar synovitis -- Inflammation of the synovial membrane close to the kneecap.

Paraproteinemias -- Disorder characterized by paraproteins in the blood including those for multiple myeloma, cryoglobulins and others. See Multiple myeloma; cryoglobulins.

Parasites -- Organisms that live within, upon or at, the expense of another living organism. Human parasites include disease-causing agents, such as amoebas or worms, that infect the digestive system or fungi that live on skin.

Parasitic disease -- Any one of many diseases caused by a parasite. See Parasites.

Parathyroids -- Small glands that control calcium levels in the blood and bones. Located within or next to the thyroid gland in the lower neck, next to the trachea.

Paresthesias -- Abnormal sensation of the skin, such as numbness, prickling and tingling, that occurs without apparent cause.

Parkinson's disease -- Disease of the central nervous system in older adults characterized by gradual, progressive muscle rigidity, tremors and clumsiness. Cause is usually unknown, although medications, brain injury, tumor or infection may cause it. Currently incurable, but treatment can control or relieve symptoms.

Paroxysmal nocturnal hemoglobinuria (PNH) -- Disorder characterized by the destruction of red blood cells resulting in hemoglobin being excreted in the urine. It occurs in irregular episodes for several days in a row, especially at night. Usually afflicts adults between 25 and 45 years of age and is accompanied by abdominal pain, back pain and headache.

Pathology laboratory -- Lab where tissues, blood, urine, feces and other parts of the human body are studied to determine cause of disease.

Pelvic inflammatory disease (P.I.D.) -- Infection of female reproductive organs. May be contagious if the infecting germ is sexually transmitted. Gonorrhea is a common cause. See Gonorrhea.

Peptic ulcer -- Lesion of the mucous membrane lining of the stomach, duodenum or of any part of the digestive tract exposed to stomach acids. See Ulcers. Acute peptic ulcers are often shallow and cause no scars or symptoms. Chronic peptic ulcers are often deep, cause scarring of the tissue and are persistent. Symptoms may include a gnawing pain, vomiting, loss of appetite and weight loss. Serious complications include bleeding, perforation and malignant change. Treatment may include antacids, medication that blocks the formation of stomach acid and diet changes.

Percutaneous -- Performed through the skin. In some procedures, a needle is passed through the skin to a space below the skin to obtain fluid or to inject a fluid, dye or medication.

Pericardial effusion -- Escape of fluid. into the pericardium. See Pericardium.

Pericarditis, acute -- Inflammation of the sac that covers the heart. Symptoms may include chest pain that worsens with movement, rapid breathing, cough, fever and chills, weakness and anxiety. Cause may be unknown. Sometimes caused by infection or as a complication of an illness or chest injury. Usually curable in 6 months unless it is caused by cancer.

Pericardium -- Thin, membranous, double-layered covering of the heart.

Periodontal disease (Periodonitis) -- Inflammation and infection of the gums, causing loss of supporting bone. Can result in tooth loss. Not contagious.

Peripheral-artery disease -- Any abnormal condition that affects the arteries outside the heart. Signs and symptoms may include numbness, pain and paleness of the involved area(s) and hypertension. See Hypertension. Causes include obesity, cigarette smoking, stress, inactive lifestyle, various metabolic disorders and emboli. See Embolism. One type is arteriosclerosis. See Arteriosclerosis.

Peripheral circulation (Peripheral vascular system) -- Network of arteries, veins and lymphatic channels supplying the head, arms and legs.

Peripheral vessels -- See Peripheral circulation.

Peritoneum -- Covering of the intestinal tract and lining of the walls of the abdominal and pelvic cavities. **Peritonitis** -- Serious infection or inflammation of part or all of the peritoneum. May be fatal if not treated promptly.

Pernicious anemia -- See Anemia, pernicious.

Petechiae -- Tiny purple or red spots that appear on the skin as a result of very minute hemorrhages. **Petit mal epilepsy** -- See Epilepsy, petit mal.

pH--Symbol expressing the acidity of alkalinity of a solution on a scale of 0 to 14. pH 7 is neutral. Above 7 is alkaline. Below 7 is acid.

Pharyngeal -- Pertaining to the pharynx or voice box in the throat, which contains the vocal cords.

Pharyngitis -- Throat inflammation and infection that can be caused by a variety of germs (bacteria, viruses, fungi). Symptoms include sore throat, difficulty swallowing, fever, body aches and sometimes swollen glands in the neck. Treatment varies depending on the type of germ causing the pharyngitis.

Phenylketonuria (PKU) -- Inherited disorder marked by the inability of phenylalanine (an amino acid) to metabolize appropriately. Results in an accumulation of phenylalanine, which is toxic to brain tissue. If left untreated, results in progressive mental retardation. Most states require a PKU screening test for all newborns. Treatment consists of a diet free of phenylalanine.

Pheochromocytoma -- Tumor of the core (medulla) of the adrenal glands. Tumor is usually benign and does not spread to other organs. See Adrenal medulla tumors.

Phlebitis -- Inflammation of a vein.

Phototherapy -- Treatment of a disease by exposure to light, especially variously concentrated light rays.

Pituitary diabetes insipidus -- Metabolic disorder due to injury of the pituitary gland causing a deficient production of anti-diuretic hormone. Patients have great thirst and pass copious amounts of urine.

Placenta previa -- Bleeding late in pregnancy caused by placenta attaching too low in the uterus, covering the cervix completely or partially. (The cervix contains the opening into the birth canal). This can be life-threatening to the unborn child and to the mother. The most common sign is sudden, painless bleeding, usually in the last trimester. With prompt care, mothers and most infants survive without complications. In some cases, delivery is necessary before the fetus is mature enough to survive. **Placental sulfatase deficiency** -- Deficiency of sulfatase in the placenta.

Plaques -- 1) Small raised area of abnormal material on a surface, such as the skin or blood vessel lining. 2) Mixture of bacteria and calcium deposited on the teeth that can cause cavities and gum disease. **Plasma** -- Fluid part of the blood after blood cells and other particles are removed.

Plasmapheresis (Therapeutic plasma exchange; TPE) -- Blood is withdrawn from a vein in the arm and passed through a cell separator to remove cells from the plasma. The blood cells are then transfused back into the individual. TPE is used to treat immune disorders.

Plasmin -- Active portion of the chemical system that causes blood clots to dissolve.

Plasminogen-activator system -- System that stimulates the conversion of chemical substances to plasmin. See Plasmin.

Platelets -- Tiny blood cells (much smaller than red or white blood cells) that assist in blood clotting. A drop of blood contains about 12.5-million platelets.

Pleura -- Thin tissue lining of the lungs and chest cavity.

Pleural -- Relating or pertaining to pleura. See Pleura.

Pleurisy -- Inflammation of the pleura. See Pleura. A painful condition caused by lung disease.

Pneumatosis cytoides intestinalis -- Disease characterized by the presence of air or gas in abnormal pockets in the intestinal tract. Usually associated with an infection.

Pneumonia -- Inflammation of the lung(s) resulting in tiny air sacs in the lung becoming plugged with exudate. Can be caused by bacteria, viruses or fungi.

Pneumonitis -- Inflammation of lung tissue that may be caused by a virus or it may be an allergic response to chemicals, dust or mold. A dry cough is a common sign. Treatment depends on the cause, but often includes the administration of corticosteroids to reduce inflammation.

Pneumothorax -- Collapse of all or part of a lung caused by pressure from free air in the chest between the two layers of the pleura. See Pleura.

Polycystic -- Containing many cysts.

Polycystic ovaries (Stein-Leventhal syndrome) -- Ovary enlargement from many small cysts. Ovary surface becomes too thick to allow ovulation. Women with this problem cannot become pregnant without treatment.

Polycythemia -- Increase in red blood cells in the body. The disease has three forms. Polycythemia vera involves overproduction of red blood cells, white blood cells and platelets. Secondary polycythemia is a complication of diseases or factors other than blood cell disorders. Stress polycythemia involves decreased blood plasma.

Polycythemia vera -- Overproduction of red blood cells, white blood cells and platelets. Cause is unknown. Treatment may include withdrawing blood at certain intervals, radioisotope therapy and drug therapy. Treatment is needed to prevent blood clots from forming that could cause a stroke, heart attack or blockage in a vein or artery.

Polymyositis -- Inflammation of many muscles at one time. Usually accompanied by muscle weakness, deformity, swelling, pain, sweating and tension. Sometimes associated with malignant conditions.

Polyneuritis -- Inflammation of many nerves simultaneously. In acute infectious polyneuritis (Guillain-Barre syndrome), inflammation of nerves and muscles progresses, rapidly causing weakness, loss of sensation and sometimes paralysis for weeks or months. Cause is unknown, but it sometimes follows an infection, immunization or minor surgery. May be an autoimmune disorder.

Polyposis -- Formation of numerous polyps. See Polyps. Familial polyposis is an inherited condition in which the intestinal lining contains many polyps, some of which are highly likely to become malignant. **Polyps** -- Growths. Often on a stalk arising from dry mucous membranes, such as in the nose, cervix or colon.

Porphyria -- Excretion of porphyrins into the urine. See Porphyrins.

Porphyria, acute intermittent (AIP) -- Rare inherited disorder characterized by excessive formation and excretion of porphyrins. See Porphyrins. Symptoms include recurrent abdominal pain often accompanied by nausea, vomiting, constipation and dark urine.

Porphyria cutanea tarda -- Type of porphyria usually associated with chronic alcoholism marked by skin lesions and enlarged liver. See Porphyria, acute intermittent.
Porphyrins -- Any of a group of pyrrole derivatives found in cytoplasm. These combine with iron and magnesium to form other substances.
Portacaval shunt -- Connection of the portal vein with the vena cava to release backed-up pressure in the veins that drain the intestinal tract.
Portal hypertension -- Higher than normal blood pressure in the large vein that collects nourishment from intestinal absorption then drains into the liver.
Post-streptococcal glomerulonephritis -- Inflammatory disease of kidney occurring about 3 weeks following a strep infection elsewhere in the body. Probably related to an effect on body's immune system. **Pott's disease (Tuberculous spondylitis)** -- Rare, grave form of tuberculosis that is located in the spinal column. See Tuberculosis. Segments of the spine may actually collapse. Symptoms include stiffness and painfulness of the spine. Abscesses may form and put pressure on the spinal cord, resulting in areas of paralysis.
Precocious puberty -- Changes of adolescence that occur sooner than expected in young girls or boys.
Pre-eclampsia (Toxemia of pregnancy) -- Serious disturbance in blood pressure, kidney function and the central nervous system that may occur from the 20th week of pregnancy until 7 days after delivery. Not accompanied by seizures. See Eclampsia.
Primary biliary cirrhosis -- Disease of the liver caused from chronic bile retention. Cause is unknown. See Cirrhosis.
Primary hypothyroidism -- Overabundance of aldosterone, a hormone produced and secreted by the adrenal gland.
Primary lymphedema -- Chronic swelling of a part due to the accumulation of fluid (lymph) caused by obstruction of lymph vessels. Primary lymphedema may be congenital or caused by abnormal increase in number of cells of lymph vessels.
Proctitis -- Inflammation of the rectum and tissues around the anus. Can be caused by sexually transmitted infections, other infections, cancer of the rectum, food allergies or chronic constipation. Usually curable with appropriate treatment specific to the cause.
Profile -- Most hospital and commercial laboratories offer blood tests collected together in PACKAGES (sometimes called profiles). The number of tests in each package and the cost varies between laboratories. On your bill, a sum is usually quoted for the entire package of tests, without breaking out the charge for each test. In the lab report, the result and name of each test are clearly marked. Some common profiles include coronary risk profile, electrolyte package, hepatitis profile, liver profile, thyroid profile and chemical profile. Each is covered in this glossary.
Prolonged activiated partial thromboplastin time -- Longer-than-normal time required for clotting to take place in the activated thromboplastin time test.
Prostate -- Gland surrounding the neck of the bladder and urethra in men.
Prostatic hypertrophy -- Enlargement of the prostate. See Prostate. May obstruct the flow of urine from the bladder. Not cancerous. Symptoms may include urinary urgency and frequency, burning on urination, weak urinary stream, a feeling that the bladder cannot be emptied and sometimes impotence. Curable with surgery.
Prostatitis -- Inflammation or infection of the prostate. See Prostate. Not contagious. Symptoms may include urinary urgency and frequency, burning on urination, difficulty starting urination and emptying bladder completely, fever, chills, pain in scrotum, anus or lower back, and muscle or joint aches. Usually curable with treatment, which includes antibiotics.
Protein metabolism -- Process by which protein foods are used by the body to make tissue proteins, together with breaking down tissue proteins to produce energy. Food proteins are first broken down into amino acids then absorbed into the blood and finally used in body cells to form new proteins. Diseases affecting protein metabolism include liver disease, maple-sugar urine disease and phenylketonuria. See Maple-sugar urine disease; phenylketonuria.
Proteus infections -- Bacteria normally found in feces, water and soil. May cause urinary tract

infections, kidney infections, wound infections, diarrhea and bacteremia. See Bacteremia.
Pseudocysts -- Abnormal or dilated space resembling a cyst but without a membrane lining. Condition commonly occurs after pancreatitis. See Pancreatitis. Surgery may be required to drain pseudocysts. **Pseudogout** -- Arthritic condition marked by attacks of gout-like symptoms, usually affecting a single joint (particularly the knee). Inflammation and pain may be relieved by hydrocortisone injections into the affected joint or by taking antiinflammatory medications.
Pseudohypoparathyroidism -- Hereditary condition that resembles hypoparathyroidism. In hypoparathyroidism, there is a deficiency of parathyroid hormone. In pseudohypoparathyroidism, there is no deficiency of hormone, but the body fails to respond normally to the parathyroid hormone. Symptoms may include short stature, crossed eyes, calcium deposits in muscle and brain tissue, and mental retardation.
Pseudomembranous enterocolitis (Necrotizing enterocolitis) -- Acute inflammatory bowel disorder that usually occurs in premature or low-birth-weight newborns. Cause is unknown. Characterized by death of tissue of the intestinal walls, which may lead to perforation and peritonitis. See Peritonitis. Early symptoms may include low body temperature, poor feeding, vomiting and blood in stools. Without treatment, death is likely.
Pseudo-precocious puberty -- Premature sexual development; of unknown cause. **Pseudotumors** -- False or phantom tumor.
Psoriasis -- Chronic, scaly skin disorder characterized by frequent remissions and recurrences. Affected skin areas are raised, have red borders and are covered with large, silver-white scales. Areas may crack and become painful. Treatment can control symptoms, but there is no cure.
Pulmonary -- Lungs.
Pulmonary disease -- Lung disease.
Pulmonary edema -- Accumulation of fluid in the lungs. Caused by a failing heart.
Pulmonary embolism -- Blood clot or fat cells (rarely) in one of the arteries carrying blood to the lungs. Blood clot begins in a deep vein of the leg or pelvis. Fat embolus usually begins at a fracture site. Embolus moves through the blood, passing through the heart and lodging in the branch of an artery that nourishes the lungs. This blockage decreases breathing ability and sometimes destroys lung tissue. **Pulmonary fibrosis** -- Fibrous tissue in the lungs causing scarring of tissue from one of many disease processes, such as emphysema.
Pulmonary infarctions -- Death of a section of lung tissue from obstruction of the blood supply. See Pulmonary embolism.
Pulmonary insufficiency -- Subnormal function of the lungs.
Pulmonary valve -- Separates the right bottom chamber of the heart (ventricle) from the pulmonary artery (the large artery that goes from the heart to the lungs).
Pulmonary-valve stenosis -- Narrowing of the pulmonary valve. Impairs heart function. Usually there are no symptoms at first. As the condition worsens, chest pain, dizziness, faintness upon exertion and congestive heart failure symptoms develop. When symptoms become severe, surgery is recommended to stretch the defective pulmonary valve. See Congestive heart failure.
Purines -- Any of a large group of nitrogen compounds. End products after digestion of certain proteins; also made by the body. Present in many medications and in some foods.
Purpura -- Purplish or brownish discoloration easily seen through the skin caused by bleeding into the tissues.
Pyelonephritis (Kidney infection) -- Noncontagious bacterial infection of the kidneys. Infection may begin in the bladder and ascend to the kidneys. May be acute or chronic. Acute infections come on rapidly and are often characterized by fever, chills, nausea, flank pain and urinary frequency and burning. Antibiotic therapy usually cures the infection in 10 to 14 days. Chronic infections develop slowly and last for months or years. They lead to scarring and eventual loss of kidney function. If chronic kidney failure develops in both kidneys, kidney transplant or kidney dialysis can be life saving.
Pyloric stenosis -- Condition in infancy in which encircling muscles enlarge and cause obstruction. It occurs in infants, usually beginning at 2 to 5 weeks. Causes projectile vomiting after feedings.

Pyridoxine-responsive anemia -- See Anemia, pyridoxine-responsive.

R INDEX

Radiation therapy (Radiotherapy) -- Use of high-energy waves, generated by special X-ray machines, cobalt machines and other devices, to treat some forms of cancer. Radiation destroys cancerous tissue, but does little harm to healthy tissue.

Radiography -- Making X-ray films of internal structures of the body by exposure of film specially sensitized to X-rays or gamma rays.

Radioisotope -- Radioactive form of chemical normally present in the body. Chemical elements that give off radiation. A radioisotope of a chemical element normally present in the body, such as carbon, will mix with non-isotopes when it is injected into the body.

Radioisotope scan -- Radioisotope is given orally or intravenously and becomes concentrated in organs, such as the heart, lungs or brain. Instruments measure the radiation given off by the radioisotopes and create a photographic image of the organ being studied. See Radioisotope.

Radiotherapy -- See Radiation therapy.

Raynaud's disease -- Primary disorder of the circulatory system that affects blood circulation to fingers and occasionally toes. Occurs mostly in people who smoke. This is different from Raynaud's phenomenon, which occurs as a complication of other diseases.

Raynaud's phenomenon -- Circulation system disorder affecting fingers and toes. A complication of an underlying disease or emotional disturbance. This is different from Raynaud's disease. See Raynaud's disease.

Rebound stimulation -- Response is reversed when stimulus is withdrawn.

Red cell indices -- Blood test that provides important information about the size, hemoglobin concentration and hemoglobin weight of an average blood cell. Aids in classification of anemias. Indices include mean corpuscular volume (MCV), mean corpuscular hemoglobin (MCH) and mean corpuscular hemoglobin concentration (MCHC). MCV expresses the average size of many cells and indicates whether most red blood cells are undersized (microcytic), oversized (macrocytic) or normal sized (normocytic). MCH is the hemoglobin-to-red-blood-cell ratio and gives the weight (concentration) of hemoglobin in an average red blood cell. MCHC defines the volume of hemoglobin in an average red cell and helps distinguish normally colored (normochromic) red blood cells from pale (hypochromic) red cells.

Red measles (Rubeola) -- Serious viral disease of childhood. Uncommon today because immunizations have controlled this problem to a great extent in North America and Europe. **Reflux esophagitis** -- Irritation of the esophagus from stomach acid splashing upward into the esophagus.

Reiter's disease -- Inflammatory disease caused by symptoms resembling those of arthritis, urethritis, conjunctivitis and psoriasis. See Arthritis; urethritis; conjunctivitis; psoriasis.

Renal -- Pertaining to the kidney.

Renal disease -- Any of several diseases affecting the kidneys.

Renal plasma flow -- Rate of blood flow through the kidney.

Renal tubular acidosis -- Loss of base or accumulation of acid in the body due to disease of the kidney tubules.

Renal tubular disease -- Disease of the kidney tubules.

Renovascular hypertension (Portal hypertension) -- Abnormally high blood pressure within the vessels of portal circulation. Caused by compression or obstruction of a blood vessel(s) decreasing blood flow in this area. The portal circulation system is a network of veins that carries blood from abdominal organs to the liver. Portal hypertension is frequently associated with alcoholic cirrhosis, but also results from blood clots in the hepatic (liver) or portal vein, constrictive pericarditis or a defective tricuspid valve in the heart. Portal hypertension results in an enlarged spleen and ascites, and in severe cases, generalized high blood pressure and esophageal varices. See Cirrhosis; hypertension; ascites; esophageal varices.

Restrictive pericarditis -- Pressure develops when an increasing amount of fluid restricts the pumping action of the heart. Caused by development of fluid between the heart and the sac covering the heart. Treatment may include medication, aspiration of fluid from the sac using a needle or surgery to remove fluid from the sac. See Pericarditis.

Reticulocytes -- Young, immature red blood cells.

Reticulocytosis -- Excess amount of reticulocytes in the blood.

Reticuloendothelial system -- Body system involved primarily in defense against infection and in disposal of products of the breakdown of cells. Made up of cells that are able to surround, engulf and digest microorganisms and cell debris (macrophages) and special cells in the liver, lungs, bone marrow, spleen and lymph nodes.

Retina -- Innermost part of the eyeball.

Retinitis pigmentosa -- Hereditary disease marked by progressive loss of retinal response, leading to partial or total blindness.

Retinopathy -- Any non-inflammatory disease of the retina. Associated with various conditions. It is most frequently seen in people with untreated hypertension or with diabetes mellitus. See Hypertension; diabetic retinopathy.

Retroperitoneal -- Pertaining to organs closely attached to the abdominal wall, behind the peritoneum. **Retroperitoneal thrombosis** -- Clotting of blood in the retroperitoneal space.

Reye's syndrome -- Disease in children and adolescents that involves brain and other major organs. Can cause permanent brain damage, coma or death due to pressure on brain. With treatment, most children survive and recover completely. Aspirin has been linked to influenza and various viral diseases as a possible cause. Children with influenza or chickenpox should not be given aspirin to reduce fever! **Rh-factor** -- Symbol for rhesus factor. Antigens present on the surface of red blood cells. **Rh-isoimmunization** -- Development of agglutination against Rh-blood group antigens in an Rh-negative person in response to Rh-positive blood. It may lead to serious or fatal reactions to blood transfusion or development of erythroblastosis fetalis in the fetus of a subsequent pregnancy. See Agglutination; erthyroblastosis fetalis.

Rheumatic fever -- Inflammatory complication of Group-A strepococcal infections that affects many parts of the body, especially joints and the heart. Strep infections are contagious, but rheumatic fever is not.

Rheumatoid arthritis -- Illness characterized by joint disease that involves muscles, cartilage and membrane linings of the joints. Three times more common in women than men. Symptoms include red, warm, painful joints. Sometimes accompanied by weakness and fatigue. If disease is severe, permanent deformity and crippling may result.

Rickets -- Condition caused by insufficient intake or absorption of vitamin D coupled with too little exposure to sunlight. Seen primarily in infants and small children. Characterized by abnormal bone formation. Symptoms include soft, pliable bones, enlarged skull, muscle pain and profuse sweating.

Rickettsial-collagen disease -- Connective tissue disease caused by rickettsial germs. **Rickettsial disease** -- Any disease caused by rickettsial microorganisms. Transmitted to humans by bites from infected lice, fleas, ticks and mites. Rickettsial diseases have been responsible for some of the worst epidemics in history.

Rickettsial germs -- Microorganisms smaller than bacteria and larger than viruses. Cause various diseases.

Ring-chromosome formation -- Chromosome in which both ends have been lost; broken ends have reunited to form a ring-shaped figure.

Rocky Mountain spotted fever -- Caused by rickettsial germs transmitted by a tick bite. Symptoms include high fever, headache, body aches and skin rash. Tongue is covered with a thick, white coating that turns brown as the fever persists and rises. Fatal disease in 5% of those infected, especially anyone who delays treatment or is older. Incidence is increasing as camping and backpacking become more popular outdoor activities. See Rickettsial disease.

Rubella (German measles) -- Mild, contagious viral illness. Likely to cause serious birth defects to an unborn baby of a pregnant woman who develops the disease in the first 3 or 4 months of pregnancy.

Symptoms of mother-to-be include fever, muscle aches, stiff neck, fatigue, headache, reddish rash that develops on the second or third day of illness and lasts only 1 to 2 days, and swollen lymph glands in the neck. Spontaneous recovery occurs in 1 week in children, longer in adults.

S INDEX

Salivary-gland disease -- Disease of the salivary glands, which secrete saliva.

Salmonella -- Thousands of kinds of salmonella bacteria cause many diseases, including typhoid fever, paratyphoid fever and some forms of gastroenteritis (inflammation of the stomach and intestines). **Salt-losing syndrome** -- Condition characterized by vomiting, dehydration, abnormally low blood pressure and even sudden death due to very large sodium losses from the body. Can occur due to large sodium loss from the gastrointestinal tract or from excessive sodium loss into the urine (as in congenital adrenal hyperplasia or adrenocortical insufficiency). See Adrenal hyperplasia.

Sandhoff's disease -- Variant of Tay-Sachs disease that has a progressive, more rapid course. Found in the general population. Tay-Sachs disease usually only affects Ashkenazic Jewish infants. See Tay-Sachs disease.

Sarcoidosis -- Chronic, progressive disease of unknown cause. May cause symptoms in the skin, lungs, lymph nodes, liver, spleen, eyes and bones of the hands and feet. No specific treatment.

Sarcoma -- Tumor derived from connective tissue.

Scan -- Shortened form of scintiscan, a diagnostic procedure using a scintillation camera to record images of various parts of the body following injection of appropriate radioactive substances. This is a major tool for establishing precise diagnoses.

Scarlatina (Scarlet fever) -- Childhood disorder characterized by a bright-red rash. Scarlet fever is preceded by a streptococcal throat infection. Both are very contagious.

Scarlet fever -- See Scarlatina.

Scleroderma -- Widespread connective tissue disease in which skin and other body parts gradually degenerate, thicken and become stiff. See Connective tissue disease.

Sclerosing cholangitis -- Scarring and inflammation of a bile duct.

Scoliosis -- Abnormal lateral curve of a normally straight spine.

Scotoma -- Area of depressed or decreased vision in the visual field that is surrounded by an area of normal (or less depressed) vision.

Scurvy (Vitamin-C deficiency) -- Illness caused by inadequate intake of vitamin C. Vitamin C is essential for the body to manufacture connective tissue (collagen) that helps form healthy bones, teeth and capillaries, and promotes wound healing. Symptoms in children may include tender, swollen legs, bleeding and bruising under the skin, bleeding gums, fever and anemia. See Anemia. Adults may have swollen, bleeding gums, tooth loss, bleeding or bruising under the skin or bleeding into joints, weakness and mental changes. Treatment includes a balanced diet and vitamin-C supplementation. All symptoms, except tooth loss, are reversible.

Seborrheic dermatitis -- Skin condition characterized by greasy or dry, white scales. Dandruff and cradle cap are both forms of seborrheic dermatitis. Not contagious.

Secondary hypothyroidism -- Low thyroid function from drugs or other cause.

Secondary lymphedema -- Swelling of a body part due to the accumulation of fluid caused by inflammation, obstruction or removal of lymph vessels. May follow mastectomy surgery when breast tissue and lymph vessels are removed. Obstruction of lymph vessels may be caused by malignant tumors or infestation with adult filiarial parasites. See Filariasis.

Secondary syphilis -- Second stage of syphilis, characterized by skin rash, fever, swollen glands and headache. See Syphilis.

Sella turcica -- Depression in the floor of the skull that contains the pituitary gland.

Sensorineuraly deafness -- Loss of hearing due to a lesion in the acoustic nerve (the eighth cranial nerve).

Septal defects -- Abnormal, usually congenital, defect in the wall separating two chambers of the heart. **Septic arthritis** -- Infection in any joint in the body. See Arthritis.

Serous -- Pertaining to or resembling serum. See Serum.

Serum -- Liquid portion of the blood that remains after blood cells have been removed.
Serum sickness -- Hypersensitivity reaction following administration of an antiserum. Characterized by fever, hives, swollen lymph glands, joint pain and enlarged spleen.
Sexual precocity -- Attainment of sexual maturity before the 6th birthday in girls and the 8th birthday in boys. This is an abnormal condition. Sexual development follows the usual pattern of normal puberty except the child's psychological sexuality is not mature. Cause is usually unknown. Sometimes caused by tumors of the hypothalamus or pineal gland. Other causes include Albright syndrome and untreated juvenile hypothyroidism.
Shigellosis -- Dysentery produced by an infection by a shigella germ. **Sickle cell anemia** -- See Anemia, sickle cell.
Sickle cell trait -- Anemia and other signs of sickle cell anemia do not occur in the person with sickle cell trait. People who have the trait are informed and counseled regarding the possibility of having an infant with sickle cell disease if both parents carry the trait. See Anemia, sickle cell.
Sigmoid -- Portion of the large intestine located in the left side of the abdomen. It connects to the descending colon above and the rectum below.
Sigmoid torsion -- Twisting of the sigmoid portion of the large intestine.
Single-vessel disease -- Disease involving only one of the coronary artery vessels. See Coronary artery disease.
Sinusitis -- Inflammation or infection of the sinuses. Usually refers to the eight sinuses adjacent to the nose.
Sjogren's disease -- See Sjogren's syndrome.
Sjogren's syndrome -- Benign, chronic inflammation that results in diminished production of tears and saliva. Cause is unknown, but it is usually associated with rheumatoid arthritis or collagen vascular disease. See Rheumatoid arthritis; collagen vascular disease.
Snellen chart -- One of several charts used to test vision. Letters, numbers or symbols are arranged on the chart in decreasing size from top to bottom.
Solid tumors -- Growth of tissue of hard, unyielding substance. Differs from a tumor filled with fluid, such as a cystic tumor.
Specificity -- Quality or state of being specific. Usually refers to restriction of effect to a particular function.
Spherocytes -- Abnormally shaped red blood cells. Cells are sphere shape, in contrast to the doughnut shape of normal red blood cells.
Spherocytosis -- Presence of spherocytes in the blood. Caused by some anemias. See Anemia. **Sphincter of Oddi** -- Sphincter muscle of the bile duct.
Spina bifida -- Inherited defective closure of the body encasement of the spinal cord through which the cord and meninges may protrude.
Spleen -- Large organ on the left side of the upper abdominal cavity next to the stomach. Helps modify the structure of the blood.
Splenectomy (Spleen removal) -- Removal of the spleen due to injury (causing rupture and uncontrolled bleeding), various blood diseases, benign or malignant tumors or a clot in the splenic vein. **Spondylolisthesis** -- Forward displacement of one vertebra upon another, usually the fifth lumbar over the body of the sacrum or of the fourth lumbar over the fifth.
Sprue -- Chronic disorder resulting from malabsorption of nutrients from the small intestine. It occurs in tropical and nontropical forms. See Tropical sprue; celiac disease.
Staphylococcemia -- Infection caused by staphylococcus bacteria in the blood. May result in endocarditis, meningitis or osteomyelitis. See Meningitis; osteomyelitis.
Staphylococcus aureus -- Bacteria that frequently causes diseases of the skin and other organs. **Steatorrhea** -- Fatty stools.
Stein-Leventhal syndrome -- See Polycystic ovaries.
Stenosis -- Narrowing or stricture of any hollow structure, such as a blood vessel or bile duct. **Stones** -- Hard, unyielding substances. Stones may be made in the liver, gallbladder, blood vessels or

urinary tract.

Storage-pool disease -- Metabolic disorder in which some substance accumulates in unusually large amounts.

Streptococcus pneumoniae -- Pneumonia from streptoccocal infection.

Streptokinase treatment -- Treatment with streptokinase to dissolve blood clots in hollow blood vessels.

Stress incontinence -- Involuntary loss of urine in women that accompanies any action that suddenly increases pressure within the abdomen, such as lifting, sneezing, singing or laughing. Treatment may include exercises to strengthen the muscles of the pelvic floor or, if severe, surgery may be required. **Stricture** -- Abnormal narrowing of a passage in the body. See Stenosis.

Strip-chart recorder -- Device that prints changes in electrical activity for measurement, such as EKG or tonometry.

Stroke (Cerebrovascular accident; CVA) -- Sudden decrease in the blood supply to part of the brain, damaging the area so it cannot function normally. Decreased blood flow can be caused by a narrowed or closed-off artery, a blood clot or other embolus blocking the blood vessel, bleeding into the brain due to a ruptured blood vessel or rupture of an aneurysm in the brain. See Embolus; aneurysm. Symptoms may include inability to speak, inability to move part of the body, uncoordination of certain muscles, headache, vision disturbance, loss of consciousness, confusion, loss of bowel and bladder control. Complete recovery is possible, but often permanent damage and disability or death occur. **Subacute bacterial endocarditis (SBE)** -- Chronic bacterial infection of the heart valves often caused by streptococcus or staphylococcus bacteria. Characterized by a slow, quiet onset, with fever, heart murmur, enlarged spleen and development of clumps of abnormal tissue (vegetations) on the flaps of a valve. Infected vegetations can break off and become an embolus. See Embolus.

Subacute hereditary tyrosinemia -- Metabolic disorder characterized by an excess of tyrosine in the blood.

Subacute thyroiditis -- Inflammation of the thyroid gland usually following mumps, influenza or other viral illness. See Mumps; influenza. Symptoms include an enlarged thyroid gland (usually 2 to 3 days after the onset of fever), body aches and malaise. Thyroid may be painful, and you may have difficulty swallowing. Treatment may include medication to relieve pain and decrease inflammation. Thyroid hormone replacement may be needed if the condition lasts more than a few days.

Subluxations -- Incomplete or partial dislocation.

Sympathomimetics -- Drugs that mimic the effects of the sympathetic nervous system, such as adrenalin and phenylephrine.

Syndrome -- Set of symptoms that occur together.

Syndrome of inappropriate anti-diuretic hormone -- See Diabetes insipidus.

Synovitis -- Inflammation or infection of the synovium. See Synovium.

Synovium -- Thick fluid secreted by a thin membrane surrounding a joint.

Syphilis -- Contagious, sexually transmitted disease that causes widespread tissue destruction if not treated promptly. Syphilis is called the great mimic because its symptoms resemble those of many other diseases.

Syphilis, late -- Final, destructive stage of the disease. Symptoms can occur anywhere from 1 to 35 years after initial infection.

Syphilis, primary -- First stage of sexually transmitted infectious syphilis. Develops approximately 3 weeks after initial contact. Characterized by the eruption of one or more chancres (small, painless, fluid-filled lesions), usually on the genitals.

Syphilis, secondary -- Develops 1 to 8 weeks after the initial chancre appears. It is characterized by a body rash. Symptoms often include headache, malaise, loss of appetite, sore throat and slight fever. **Syringomelia** -- Condition characterized by abnormal cavities filled with liquid in the spinal cord. **Systemic lupus erythematosus** -- See Lupus erythematosus, systemic.

T INDEX

TRH (Thyrotropin-releasing factor) -- Chemical substance secreted by the hypothalamus. Regulates secretion of thyroid-stimulating hormone (TSH) by the pituitary gland.

TSH (Thyroid-stimulating hormone) -- Chemical substance secreted by the pituitary gland; controls the release of thyroid hormone from the thyroid gland. TSH is needed for normal thyroid growth and function.

Tachycardia -- Heartbeat that is too fast.

Tay-Sachs disease -- Inherited, rare disorder of the central nervous system in infants and young children. It causes progressive impairment and early death. Less than 100 children are born with the disease each year in the U.S. See Sandhoff's disease.

Temporal lobe epilepsy -- See Epilepsy, temporal lobe.

Teratoma -- Tumor made up of several types of different tissue, none of which is native to the area in which it occurs. Most often found in ovaries and testes.

Thalassemia (Mediterranean anemia; hereditary leptocytosis) -- Inherited form of anemia in which red blood cells contain less hemoglobin than normal.

Thrombocytopenia -- Reduction of platelets in the blood, which reduces blood clotting and increases the risk of bleeding.

Thrombocytosis -- Abnormal increase in the number of platelets. Often causes no symptoms. Usually occurs following removal of the spleen or with hemolytic anemias, hemorrhage or iron deficiency. May also occur in advanced cancer, Hodgkin's disease or other lymphomas. See Anemia, hemolytic; Hodgkin's disease; lymphoma.

Thrombophlebitis (superficial) -- Inflammation and small blood clots in a vein near the body surface. Usually caused by infection or injury. Often occurs in the legs. This type of inflammation seldom causes clots to break loose and flow in the bloodstream, as does deep-vein thrombosis. Symptoms include hardness of the vein involved (feels like a cord), redness and tenderness in the affected area, and sometimes fever. Usually curable in 2 weeks with rest, elastic bandages on affected leg and medication to relieve inflammation and pain.

Thrombosis -- Blood clot in a blood vessel.

Thrombosis, venous (Deep-vein thrombosis) -- Blood clot that forms in a vein, usually in the lower leg or lower abdomen. It may partially or completely block blood flow or break off and travel to the lung. This is different from clots in superficial veins, which rarely break off. Symptoms include swelling and pain in the area and swelling of any part below the clot. Requires hospitalization for bed rest, observation and anti-coagulation therapy.

Thrush -- Infection by yeast cells of the mouth, usually in infants. **Thymectomy** -- Surgical removal of the thymus gland.

Thyroid profile -- Cost is about $30.00. Blood tests performed include T3 uptake and T4 uptake. See page 194. See Profile.

Thyroiditis -- Inflammation of the thyroid gland. Acute thyroiditis is caused by a bacterial infection and often results in formation of abscesses. Subacute thyroiditis usually follows a viral infection and is characterized by sore throat, fever, weakness and a painful, enlarged thyroid gland. Autoimmune thyroiditis is a chronic inflammation that can lead to Grave's disease (hyperthyroidism) or hypothyroidism if the thyroid gland diminishes in size. See Grave's disease; hypothyroidism.

Thyroxine-binding globulin abnormalities -- Condition in which abnormal globulins circulating in the blood attach to thyroxin, one hormone made by the thyroid gland.

Tibio-fibular disease -- Disorders of the two big bones of the leg between the knee and ankle. **Titer** -- Quantity of a substance required to produce a reaction with a given volume of another substance.

Tonsillitis -- Inflammation of the tonsils. Tonsils are small at birth, enlarge during childhood and become smaller at puberty. When not infected, tonsils help keep infection in the sinuses, mouth and throat from spreading to other body parts. Tonsillitis is contagious.

Tonsils -- Clumps of lymphoid tissue at the back of the throat.

Toxemia -- Presence of toxins in the bloodstream. Also called blood poisoning. See Eclampsia; pre-eclampsia.

Toxic adenoma -- Small, benign nodule in the thyroid gland that secretes thyroid hormone. Cause is unknown. Second most common cause of hyperthyroidism. Symptoms are the same as those in Grave's disease except there is no protrusion of the eyes. See Grave's disease.

Toxic nodular goiter -- Tumor of the thyroid gland with nodules. Causes overactivity of the thyroid gland.

Toxicosis -- Any disease condition due to poisoning.

Toxic-shock syndrome -- Disease characterized by sudden onset of fever, diarrhea, vomiting, sore throat, aching muscles, falling blood pressure and skin rash on palms and soles of the feet. Has been reported most often as occurring in women who use super-absorbent tampons during menstrual periods. The germ that causes the disease is normally found in the nose, mouth and vagina.

Toxins -- Poisons, usually produced by or occurring in a microorganism.

Transferase deficiency -- Deficiency of any group of enzymes called transferase. Transferase enzymes catalyze the transfer from one molecule to another of a chemical group that does not exist in a free state during the transfer.

Transferrin -- Substance present in the blood. It is essential for transportation of iron from the intestine into the blood. It makes iron available to the bone marrow, where red blood cells are produced. **Transient ischemic attacks (TIA)** -- Temporary decrease in blood supply to part of the brain. The affected part of the brain is temporarily unable to function normally.

Translocation -- Removal to another place. In genetics, the shifting of a segment or fragment of one chromosome into another part.

Tricuspid regurgitation -- Abnormal flow of blood backward through the tricuspid valves. **Tricuspid stenosis** -- Closure of the tricuspid valves.

Tricuspid valves -- Valves between the left ventricle and the aorta.

Tri-Iodothyronine (T3 3) toxicosis (Thyroid storm) -- Crisis in uncontrolled hyperthyroidism caused by the release of too much thyroid hormone. Thyroid storm may be preceded by infection or stress, or it may occur spontaneously. Also may occur after surgical removal of the thyroid gland (thyroidectomy). Characterized by high fever, up to 106F (41C), rapid pulse, severe difficulty breathing, fear, restlessness, irritability and exhaustion. The person may become delirious, lapse into a coma and die of heart failure.

Triploidy -- Presence in humans of 69 chromosomes (3 full sets). Frequently causes miscarriages. **Trisomy** -- Addition of a third chromosome to an otherwise normal cell.

Trochar -- Instrument with a blunt component inside a sharp tube. Used to pierce the wall of a body cavity, such as the chest or abdomen.

Tropical sprue -- Chronic form of malabsorption accompanied by diarrhea; occurs in the tropics and subtropics.

Tuberculosis -- Contagious, bacterial infection caused by the germ mycobacterium tuberculosis. Usually affects the lungs, but may spread to other organs.

Tubular epithelial damage -- Damage to the lining cells of kidney tubules. **Tubular function** -- Normal function of kidney tubules.

Tularemia -- Infectious bacterial disease of rodents that is transmissible to man by infected insects or direct contact. Symptoms include fever, headache, pneumonia, ulcerations in the digestive tract or ulcers on the skin, depending on the site of entry into the body. See Pneumonia; ulcers. Treatment includes antibiotics.

Tumor -- New growth of tissue in which multiplication of cells is uncontrolled and progressive.

Turner's syndrome -- Chromosome abnormality seen in about 1 in 3,000 live female births. It is marked by the absence of one sex chromosome. Characterized by short stature, primary amenorrhea and lack of development of secondary sex characteristics. Other features, which may or may not occur, include webbed neck, lowset ears, broad shield-like chest, hypertension, heart abnormalities and learning disorders. Treatment includes hormone therapy. See Amenorrhea; hypertension.

Typhus -- Disease caused by various species of rickettsia. Symptoms include fever, chills, headache, malaise and a skin rash. See Rickettsial disease.

U INDEX

Ulcer -- Round, crater-like lesion of the skin or mucous membrane resulting from tissue death. Accompanies some inflammatory, infectious or cancerous conditions.

Ulcerative colitis -- Serious, chronic inflammatory disease of the large intestine (colon). Characterized by ulceration and episodes of bloody diarrhea. Ulcerated areas are inflamed and may form abscesses in the lining of the colon.

Unconjugated bilirubin -- Fat-soluble form of bilirubin that circulates in loose association with plasma proteins. Also called indirect bilirubin.

Uremia -- Presence in blood of excessive amounts of protein metabolism byproducts, such as urea. Results in a toxic condition (as occurs in kidney failure) characterized by nausea, vomiting, dizziness, convulsions and coma.

Ureter -- Tube that carries urine from the kidney to the bladder.

Ureteroceles -- Prolapse of the end of the ureter where it joins the bladder. Prolapse is a falling or sliding of a part from its usual position. The condition may lead to obstruction of urine flow and result in hydronephrosis and loss of kidney function. Surgery is required to prevent permanent kidney damage. See Hydronephrosis.

Urethra -- Hollow anatomical structure that leads from the bladder to outside the body. **Urethritis** -- Inflammation or infection of the urethra.

Urogenital -- Referring to the kidney and reproductive systems of the human body. Also called genitourinary.

Urokinase treatment -- Treatment with the enzyme urokinase found in urine. Enzyme activates the system that dissolves blood clots in the body.

V INDEX

Valvular heart disease -- Complication of diseases that distort or destroy heart valves. The heart has four valves. Valvular heart disease can be narrowed valves (stenosis) that obstruct blood flow or widened or scarred valves that allow blood to leak backward into the heart (insufficiency or regurgitation). Disorder may be inherited or caused by another disease, such as rheumatic fever, hypertension, atherosclerosis, endocarditis or syphilis (rarely). Disease outcome depends on the underlying condition. Many complications and symptoms can be controlled with medication or cured with surgery. See Rheumatic fever; hypertension; syphilis.

Varices -- Enlarged veins, arteries or lymph vessels.

Vasculitis -- Inflammation of a blood vessel.

Vasoconstriction -- State in which blood vessels are tightened or narrowed. Can be caused by the nervous system sending messages to the blood vessels to constrict. Can also be induced by medications. **Vasopressin** -- Hormone made by the hypothalamus and stored in the pituitary gland. Effects include contraction of the muscular layer of small blood vessels, contraction of the smooth muscles of the intestinal tract and stimulation of contraction of the uterus. Also called anti-diuretic hormone. Has specific effect on kidney tubules stimulating resorption of water, causing a concentration of the urine. **Vasopressin-resistant diabetes insipidus** -- Diabetes insipidus that does not respond to treatment with vasopressin. See Diabetes insipidus.

Venous hypertension -- Pressure in veins that is higher than normal. **Venous thrombosis** -- Blood clot in a vein.

Vertebral-artery disease -- Disease (usually hardening of the artery) in the vertebral artery, a large artery that supplies blood to the neck, vertebrae, cerebellum and other parts of the brain and spinal cord. **Vesicoureteral reflux** -- Condition in which urine flows backward from the bladder into the ureters and kidneys. Because the bladder empties poorly, a urinary tract infection may result, possibly leading to chronic pyelonephritis and even to kidney damage. See Pyelonephritis. The reflux may be caused by a congenital defect, a bladder infection or a neurogenic bladder. Sometimes cause is unknown. Treatment includes administration of antibiotics. Rarely, surgery may be required.

Vestibular -- Pertaining to an oral cavity in the middle of the inner ear.

Virilization -- Process in which secondary male sexual characteristics are acquired by a female, usually

the result of dysfunction of the adrenal gland(s) or hormone medication. Also called masculinization. **Visual field** -- Field of vision measured by special tests.
Vitreous (Vitreous humor) -- Clear fluid that fills much of the eye.
Von Willebrand's disease -- Inherited disorder characterized by abnormally slow clotting of the blood, causing spontaneous nosebleeds or bleeding of the gums. Due to a deficiency of blood factor VIII. Excessive bleeding can also occur following surgery or during menstruation. See Hemophilia; factor VIII.

W [INDEX](#)

Waldenstrom's macroglobulinemia -- Rare, progressive disorder associated with abnormal proteins in the blood, swollen lymph glands, enlarged liver and spleen, anemia and bone marrow changes. See Anemia.
Wedging -- Crowding, forcing or pushing into a limited space.
Wegener's granulomatosis -- Progressive disease characterized by lesions in the bronchi and lungs, scarring of small arteries and widespread inflammation of all organs of the body.
Whipple's disease -- Malabsorption disease characterized by diarrhea, fat in the stool, skin pigmentation, joint diseases and lesions in the central nervous system.
Whooping cough -- Serious, contagious, bacterial infection of the bronchial tubes and lungs, most common in children.
Wilm's tumor -- Rapidly developing malignant tumor of the kidneys in children under 5 years of age. **Wilson's syndrome** -- Degeneration of the liver and the nucleus of the lens in the eye.
Wiskott-Aldrich syndrome -- Inherited immunodeficiency disorder only affecting males. Characterized by severe bleeding, eczema, recurrent infections and an increased risk of developing malignancy. Causes early death with an average life span of 4 years.
Wolff-Parkinson-White syndrome -- Intermittent rapid heartbeat or atrial fibrillation with characteristic changes in an electrocardiogram (EEG).

X [INDEX](#)

Xanthines -- Class of drugs that stimulate the brain and smooth muscles, such as bronchial tubes and the heart. This family of drugs includes caffeine, theophylline, aminophylline and others.
Xerophthalmia -- Abnormal dryness and thickening of the mucous membrane lining of the eyelids and white part of the eye and cornea. Caused by vitamin-A deficiency or certain eye diseases.

Y [INDEX](#)

Yellow vision -- Objects appear yellow. One symptom of digitalis toxicity.

Z

Zenker's diverticulum -- Outpouching in the region where the pharynx and esophagus touch.
Zollinger-Ellison syndrome -- Syndrome with three features: severe ulcers of the stomach or small intestine, extreme hypersecretion of stomach acid and tumors of the pancreas. Can occur in children and adults. Treatment includes anti-ulcer medication, but complete surgical removal of the stomach may be required.

www.ingramcontent.com/pod-product-compliance
Lightning Source LLC
Chambersburg PA
CBHW081309180526
45170CB00007B/2631